The Intrinsic Energies of T'ai Chi Ch'uan

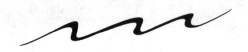

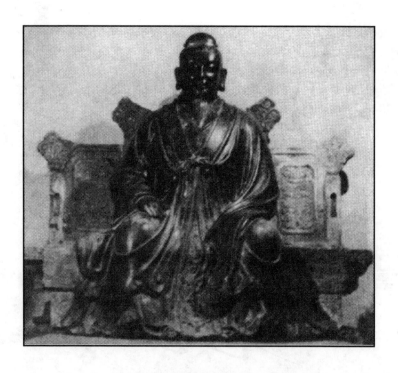

The Immortal Ancestor, Chang San-feng.
Founder of T'ai Chi Ch'uan.
A statue in his honor at Wu T'ang Temple.
Wu T'ang Mountain, Hupei Province, China.

The Intrinsic Energies
of
T'ai Chi Ch'uan

Chen Kung Series
Volume Two

Compiled and Translated by
Stuart Alve Olson

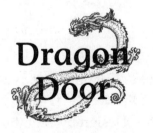

Dragon Door Publications
Saint Paul

Published by
Dragon Door Publications
Box 4381
St. Paul, Minnesota 55104 U.S.A.
(612) 645 0517

First edition (January, 1995)
Library of Congress Catalog Card Number:
ISBN : 0 938045-13-X
Cover and Interior Design by Lightbourne Images
Cover Photograph by Chris Grey, Minneapolis
Printed in the United States of America

To my wife, Lian Hwa
and our son, Lee Jin.

May the both of you
always know serasi.

Yang Family Lineage

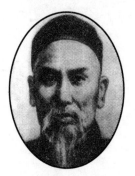

Yang Style Founder
Yang Lu-chan
(1799-1872)

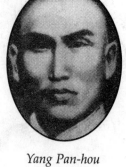

Yang Pan-hou
(1837-1892)
Eldest Son

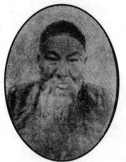

Yang Chien-hou
(1839-1917)
Second Son

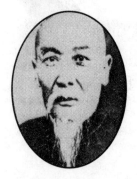

Yang Shao-hou
(1862-1930)
Eldest Son
of Yang Chien-hou

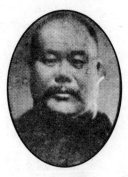

Yang Cheng-fu
(1883-1936)
Third Son
of Yang Chien-hou

Translator's Lineage

Yang Shao-hou
(1862-1930)

Yang Cheng-fu
(1883-1936)

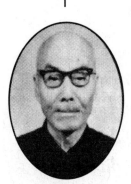

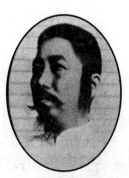

Hsiung Yang-ho
(1886-1984)

Cheng Man-ch'ing
(1901-1975)

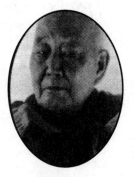

Liang Tung-tsai
(1900-)

Stuart Alve Olson
(1950-)

The poor and destitute mark your door,
hands seeking your hands.
I only brought you apples,
you gave me three bright stars.
Oh Khong Hwei,
all my efforts seem to fade,
as your ease shines on.

Acknowledgments

Without any question I could never have even attempted this book without the years of instruction and help from Master Tung-tsai Liang, as well as from his senior student Jonathan Russell. The translation work actually began nearly ten years ago. Since then I have, as Liang calls it, "mugged and bugged" him frequently about various aspects of this work. Indeed, I am very fortunate to have had him, of all the t'ai chiists in the world, to help me along with this very difficult project. I once asked Liang why no Chinese person or any of his past students had previously translated this particular section of Chen Kung's book—something which still puzzles me to this day, considering its wealth of information. He said, "Because they can't understand it. They don't know how to interpret the classics and did not study t'ai chi ch'uan extensively enough to comprehend the abstruse theories of these intrinsic energies. So young man, if you learn how to read Chinese better, then we can really talk about these things. Otherwise I can only give you a superficial understanding of these theories," Adding that I was now stealing the last piece of his art. I reminded him that it was he who first introduced me to this book by giving me a Chinese original of the text in 1982, commanding that I translate everything. He grunted in response, "dangerous cargo, I got retribution." One of his more positive approvals. Aside from his idea, I managed only to get a droplet of his art, but I will forever be in his debt for his frustrated attempts to help me understand things which were beyond mere understanding. I doubt very much, unfortunately, that I have done real justice to what we had discussed over the years. Therefore, all mistakes are mine and mine alone.

My appreciation also goes out to Dr. Poon Koonyui for providing the calligraphy that graces these pages—it is an honor to have his work included here. Calligraphy, like T'ai Chi Ch'uan, exemplifies the subtleties of intrinsic energy. Dr. Poon's work here proves that.

Very special thanks to Master Oei Khong-hwei for making very clear the theories of li and chin concerning the traditions of Shaolin boxing and T'ai Chi Ch'uan. His knowledge of these concepts are truly beyond anyone else's that I know of. I will forever be in his debt.

Much appreciation to Paul A. Crompton for his

kind words and his providing a foreword to this work.

To Fred Marych and Larry Hawkins, my sincere appreciation for taking the time to read through the original draft, for their wonderful suggestions and for helping with classes so that I could take more time to work on this book; Patrick Gross, his many suggestions, corrections and insights about the English presentation has proven quite invaluable to the final draft; John Du Cane for all his editing and format work, which in the end makes this work readable and presentable; to Vern Pererson for all his initial support of this work and friendship; to Dan Miller for providing the rare photographs of Yang Lu-chan and Yang Pan-hou, and for all his kind words of support.

Lastly, I must thank my wife Lian Hwa and her sister, Hsiang Hwa. If not for all their patient help in luring my son away from my desk and books, I fear this work would be a mere pile of torn and crumpled paper. To my son for keeping my wife busy.

The Intrinsic Energies of T'ai Chi Ch'uan

Foreword

*I*t is well nigh impossible to write an appreciation of a book such as this without having gone through all the hard work and research which the author himself has done. The next best thing is simply to acknowledge that work. From what I know, the author has had the privilege of serving a long apprenticeship with Tung-tsai Liang. This kind of experience is rare for westerners and is getting rarer still. His apprenticeship has prepared the author for producing this book.

Chinese thought and philosophy are generally expressed in short sayings, aphorisms. Such aphorisms are like small containers, ingeniously packed with a great deal of material. If you succeed in opening one of them the material may be drawn out seemingly endlessly, like the performance of a skilled conjurer. The sayings or aphorisms from which this book was translated could be the basis for writing many volumes. Thankfully, Mr. Olson has not attempted this, but has left it up to the reader to dig for himself, or herself. Likewise, his notes to the text do not try to 'better' the text but merely clarify, to the benefit of the reader.

As T'ai Chi Ch'uan deals with inner experience, the very difficult barrier of using words to describe such experience inevitably appears. When this is compounded by having to translate words from a differently structured language and an alien culture, the barrier verges on the insuperable. Mr. Olson has tackled this problem with commendable tenacity.

Paul A. Crompton

Translator's Introduction

*P*resenting this material to the general public feels both very exciting and very humbling. It is hard for a writer, especially in this relatively insignificant t'ai chi corner of the world, to provide a publication that can possibly bring more light and clarity to a subject which has already been clouded with way too much mystification. The content of this particular volume of the Chen Kung Series is, I think, a milestone within the available English literature on t'ai chi ch'uan. It has of course been available to the Chinese reader for about fifty years, and there is no question about how much has been quietly borrowed from it by Chinese t'ai chi ch'uan authors and teachers. So it is really an honor, for this "round eye," to be presenting the first English translation on this subject of intrinsic energy.

The idea of energy associated with t'ai chi ch'uan has for a number of years bordered on the mystical, and indeed at very high levels of the art this can be true, but the mainstream of t'ai chi ch'uan skills are quite available to anyone providing they practice correctly, study well and seek out reputable teachers. This work in my opinion provides many details of correct practice, will add much in the way of t'ai chi ch'uan functional theory, and act as an inspirational source for seeking out a qualified teacher.

This work covers a very broad field of t'ai chi ch'uan theory and practice. I found myself in a dilemma of sorts when adding the notes to each section of the energies. Were do I stop? In reality, each paragraph and in some cases, each sentence, deserves comment. The problem in doing so is repetition of fundamentals, as everything that is theoretical here interrelates with everything that is practical, much like the familiar problem of discussing chickens, but forever backtracking to discuss the formation of the egg. The translated text and commentary work as a whole, if you remember that nothing here is isolated from the principles of t'ai chi ch'uan. Indeed the material should be read many times to assure that you retain as much of the information as possible.

Since first publishing volume one of this series back in 1986 and the revised edition in 1993, announcing that the entire work of Chen Kung would eventually be provided in five volumes, there have been many letters of encouragement. Many thanks to those who took the time to do so. I've even heard that there are others who will also be providing English translations of certain portions of this work. I very much encourage and welcome this, as all classical material (and Chen Kung's certainly falls into that category) needs more attention than just one translation.

About the text

This volume's material comes from a section entitled, *Discourses on Intrinsic Energy*. This particular section was very difficult to translate, not because of the Chinese text, but because of the very abstruse theories presented in it. It bears repeating here, that without Tung-tsai Liang's invaluable input, this work could never have been completed. Many of the terms and theories have never previously been presented to an English audience. Additionally the work was not supported by previous translations, which is always extremely helpful when available.

The material presented here obviously represents the Yang Style point of view. I am not qualified to determine whether or not the theories and principles correspond entirely to those of the other family styles created by Chen (Wang-ting), Wu (I-hsiang), Wu (Chien-chuan), Hao (Wei-jin) and Sun (Lu-t'ang). However, we know that Yang Lu-chan studied with the Chen family for thirteen years, and that all the other styles developed from either or both of these two. It seems likely then that these theories and principles apply to all t'ai chi ch'uan styles.

The history of the text and of Chen Kung (also known as Chen Yen-lin) was given in the first volume of this series. But there are a few items which must be clarified for this volume. First, the text that Chen provides is not entirely the original. Several times Chen refers to the original text. We can only suspect why the original is not wholly reproduced. My opinion is that there were items which might be deemed unsafe or too irresponsible to present to the public at large. This I can readily understand and agree with. With the above in mind, it is also abundantly clear that Chen contributed to this particular section. There are several instances where he refers to himself in the personal, "I then ...". There are also inclusions of what Chen calls, "common sayings," which are not common by any means, quotes from ambiguous materials and stories about Yang family members. Many of these are inconsistent with the format of the text. I would guess that maybe five to ten percent of the text is Chen's creation.

The majority of the text, is undeniably, the actual work of the Yang family and even more so of their scholar-disciple, Wu Ho-ching. I would suspect that Chen Kung made some changes in order to mask the text. But this is not the work of a merchant who had studied t'ai chi ch'uan for only a few years. There is no question about the origins of the materials—they would most definitely had to have been early writings of the Yang family members and disciples. The Yang family biography provided in volume three of this series will also bear much of this out.

The text also makes reference to various other energies, such as, *tou sou* (shaking), *sung* (relaxing), *chieh* (grafting), *chuan* (rolling-up), and *che tieh* (folding up). These and a few others are not explained here, only referred to. Interestingly enough, Master Liang many years ago gave me a Chinese text written by one of his teachers, Hsiung Yang-ho, in which there are explanations of many of the missing energies referred to here. These will be presented in another work at a later date. Hsiung was a longtime and trusted disciple of Yang Shao-hou and his son Yang Chen-sheng. From the inclusion of these other energies in his book, it very might very well be possible that Hsiung had also reviewed the original text that Chen refers to. Tung-tsai Liang, who studied with Hsiung in Taiwan, feels that this is quite probable.

During the years after Shao-hou's death (1929), all students and disciples of any of the former Yang family members were ordered to become disciples of Yang Cheng-fu (Shao-hou's younger brother). But there were many who refused this edict, and actually felt insulted by it. Those who did not comply were more or less written out of Yang lineage history, which is why great masters like Chen Hsiu-feng, Chang Ching-ling, Chi Ching-chih, Hsiung Yang-ho, Li Shou-chen, and many more are virtually unheard of. Many of these disciples had skills far surpassing Yang Cheng-fu. They pointed out that Cheng-fu had not studied with his father, but was forced to learn, after his father's death, from his elder brother and other disciples of his father and uncle. Yang Cheng-fu blundered by lending out the family transcripts to Chen Yen-lin, only to have them appear publicly (which must have cost Cheng-fu a lot of face within the family). In the writings of any post Cheng-fu disciples there is no mention of any manuscripts. However, in pre Cheng-fu disciples, those who did write something, invariably explain something which is only referred to in Chen's book. It is my belief that these original manuscripts were shared, most probably in an oral manner, with trusted disciples before the Chen incident, but not after. Last question, where are these manuscripts now?

Internal energies

A frequently used statement in this text, "use the energy of the waist and legs, together with the ch'i and mind-intent," tells us that there are three aspects of *intrinsic energy*. The first is, the energy of the waist and legs, which is issued through the sinews and tendons. The second is the ch'i, issued from the spine. The third is mind-intent, issued through the will and spirit. *Chin, ch'i* and *shen* are the internal energies of the body, breath and mind. Collectively these three are referred to as *nei chin* (internal energies). Each is distinct, but at the same time a collective whole.

The treatise *The Mental Elucidation of the Thirteen Kinetic Postures* refers to these three "internal energies" in the analogy of, "The mind is the commander; the ch'i is the flag; the waist is the banner." In ancient China a commander moved his troops from one location to another during battle by sending a man with a large flag to the area first. The troops seeing the flags would then follow their men carrying banners to that location. In light of this we can view the function of these three in a couple of different manners. First. *Chin* is totally dependent upon the ch'i and shen; the ch'i need only rely on the shen and not chin; the shen need not rely on either chin or ch'i. In other words, for the chin to be issued effectively it needs the ch'i and shen; to issue ch'i effectively it needs the shen too; and, the shen can issue itself effectively without needing the chin or ch'i. Second. When the mind directs the ch'i, the waist and entire body will follow. Wherever the shen is directed, the ch'i follows, and wherever the ch'i moves, the chin will be directed.

This same treatise also says (in paraphrase), "Pay full attention to the shen, not to the ch'i [your breathing], then your striking force will be strong as pure steel. If you only pay attention to your ch'i, your blood circulation and striking force will be stagnant and ineffective." This would be akin to the flag man moving around the battle field without any direction from the commander—all the troops would scatter and the battle would be lost. However, if the flag follows the dictates of the commander, the troops will move to the proper place and the battle can be won. With this aside, we can now examine each of these three more distinctly.

Chin (intrinsic energy): the *T'ai Chi Ch'uan Treatise* says, "The energy is rooted in the feet, issued (*fa*) through the legs, directed by the waist, and appears in the hands and fingers." This is to use the energy of the waist and legs. This is also what Hsiung Yang-ho calls in his book, "The great secret of t'ai chi ch'uan application." Normally we derive strength from the upper body and limbs. T'ai chi ch'uan however derives its power from the lower body. We can understand this theory by looking at the way a whip functions. The handle of the whip is like the foot, the legs and waist resemble the length of the whip, and the hands and fingers act as the tip of the whip. Though the whip's body is soft and flowing, very strong energy is emitted from the tip.

Intrinsic energy is derived from relaxing (*sung*) the sinews and tendons. Sinews are also called chin, but this is a different ideogram. Sung is explained in note 3 of *Listening Energy*. Sinews are the parts of the flesh and muscle, elastic like young bamboo, that give strength to the muscle; tendons are the fibers which attach the flesh and muscle to the bone and bind the joints. Sinews and tendons act like rubber bands to a certain extent, and if used correctly can produce energy, just like in snapping a rubber band. And not unlike a rubber band, if stretched too far they will weaken and break; if unused they will deteriorate. But if care is taken not to go to the extreme, then the rubber band can be useful and strong. *The Mental Elucidation of the Thirteen Kinetic Postures* itself depicts the above analogy well, "only through bending and reserving will there be a surplus of intrinsic energy." The *Song of Pushing Hands* also says, "The energy appears relaxed, but is not so relaxed."

T'ai chi ch'uan exercises create blood circulation and heat (ch'i) which nourishes the sinews and tendons, strengthening their pliability and elasticity. Sung keeps the muscles and bones relaxed enough to permit the unimpeded flow of blood and ch'i through and around them. Tension obstructs the natural flow of the blood and ch'i. The principles of t'ai chi ch'uan movement and function, such as "using the body as one unit" are what allows us to issue the intrinsic energy.

Ch'i (breath and vital energy):* The classics contain numerous verses about ch'i. In *The Mental Elucidation of the Thirteen Kinetic Postures* there are two very important statements. 1) "The mind moves the ch'i. Direct the ch'i so that it sinks deeply, then it can accumulate and enter the bone. Circulate the ch'i throughout the entire body, and direct it without obstruction, so that it can easily follow the mind-intent." 2) Adhere the ch'i to the spine, allowing it to penetrate into the spine and bones." These statements refer to three important functions of ch'i cultivation: ch'i penetrating the bone, free circulation of ch'i, and the ch'i adhering to the spine.

* In order to prevent the repetition of materials relating to ch'i, it will be assumed that the reader has already reviewed the material of my book *Cultivating the Ch'i.*

The ch'i penetrates the bone. When blood and ch'i flow freely through the flesh and muscles, creating greater elasticity and pliability of the sinews and tendons, the heat (ch'i) will then affect the bone. The ch'i will permeate the bone and become marrow. Marrow has two meanings: 1) A very soft, fatty, vascular tissue of the interior cavities of the bones. 2) The essential strength and vitality of the bone. When the ch'i permeates the bones, the marrow is increased, which in turn restores and enhances the pliability of bones. As a result, the bones, as well as the sinews and tendons, acquire the energy of sung. The bones become as pliable as a baby's, but as strong as a tiger's.

Free circulation of ch'i. In t'ai chi ch'uan the concept of using ch'i meridians to circulate ch'i throughout the body is of little consequence. The idea of "free circulation" is to permeate all the bones and flesh, every minute cranny and crevice, with not only ch'i, but blood as well. This is what the Chinese call, "nourishing life" (*yang sheng*). Within the human body there are arteries, veins and corpuscles, which transport the blood throughout the entire body. Ch'i is defined as an inherent oxygen within the body. If the latent ch'i is without stimulation it will be unable to increase the flow of blood throughout the body. But if it is repeatedly stimulated it will produce heat and effectively move the blood, thus activating "free circulation." The stimulation referred to is the natural response of performing the exercises of t'ai chi ch'uan, through the regulation of breath and by letting the mind-intent direct the ch'i.

In *The Song and Substance of the Thirteen Postures* it states, "When the abdomen is completely relaxed, the ch'i will soar up and circulate throughout the entire body." *The T'ai Chi Ch'uan Classic* says, "sink the ch'i into the tan t'ien." When the stomach is relaxed the ch'i will naturally gather in the tan t'ien. Once it has gathered and has then been stimulated it will rise to circulate throughout the body.

The ch'i adheres to the spine. There are two functions of "adhering the ch'i to the spine." 1) Ch'i and breath are totally interrelated. Therefore, the inhalation is always drawn up along the spine, so that both the flow of blood increases and the ch'i permeates the spine. 2) When the ch'i begins permeating the spine this will naturally cause the entire back and shoulders to be emptied of all tension and external muscular force. This develops into intrinsic energy along the spine, just as it would in the waist and legs. Through the breath, the *ha* sound and the mind-intent, the ch'i can be issued. *The Mental Elucidation of the Thirteen Kinetic Postures* states, "The energy is issued from the spine." This means to first inhale and attract (adhere) the ch'i to the spine, which is storing or reserving energy, then at the moment of attack, issue the ch'i and intrinsic energy to the opponent.

Many t'ai chiists also practice the Taoist forms of macro-cosmic and micro-cosmic circulation of ch'i. The macro-cosmic orbit of ch'i *is* related and will aid the path of the intrinsic energy from the feet to the fingers. The micro-cosmic orbit of ch'i is also related and will aid the path of the intrinsic energy, adhering the ch'i to the spine and sinking it into the tan t'ien.

Shen (spirit and mind-intent): this is an enormously extensive subject, as it entails the whole concept of the imagination, *shen ming* (see note 5 of *Interpreting Energy*) and the more mystical aspects of Taoism. The classics contain numerous verses concerning the *shen*, which can be defined as spirit, mind, mind-intent, intention, consciousness, concentration or attention. *The Mental Elucidation of the Thirteen Kinetic Postures* says, "First in the mind, then in the body." The mind is the function, the body the substance. The body will naturally follow the dictates of the mind. To be spontaneous (*tzu jan*, or "naturally just so") means the mind need not think its way through anything, it will automatically adapt to all changes and circumstances. In the beginning you must rely on the mind, but once mastery is achieved, you can rely just on the body to react spontaneously, even without your awareness. This is the meaning of the verse in *The T'ai Chi Ch'uan Classic*, "a feather cannot be added, nor a fly can alight." The mind has made the body so sensitive and alert, that even in your sleep you cannot be attacked;

the ch'i will be circulated purely of its own accord; and, the mind will remain bright, clear and tranquil no matter the conditions.

From the t'ai chi ch'uan perspective, no opponent would dare attack someone who had attained *shen ming*. After looking into their eyes they will become confused, distracted and fearful. Even in old age someone with shen ming can physically see very far; their eyes are very bright and profoundly deep. *Shen* is expressed by the eyes; as intrinsic energy is expressed through the hands and fingers; as ch'i is expressed through the countenance of the entire body.

The *shen* is developed in t'ai chi ch'uan in three primary ways:
1) The use of imagination, which is presuming an opponent when performing the solo form of t'ai chi ch'uan. This presuming must be done with a violence-free, playful mind. The opponent is never hurt or injured, just playfully repelled or knocked down. This will help alleviate tension in both the body and mind, and also will enable you to be calm in a real attack situation (which is absolutely essential for t'ai chi ch'uan to be functional). 2)Through keeping the spine centered and upright; through drawing in the *wei lu*; and, through retaining a light and sensitive energy on top of the head, so that the spirit and vitality will be caused to rise up from the upper tan t'ien, which is the

point of the "third eye", up into the *pai hui* point on top of the head.

3) By constantly cultivating tranquillity of mind. Seek stillness within movement; seek movement within stillness. This is what the *T'ai Chi Ch'uan Treatise* means by "calmly stimulate the ch'i, with the spirit and vitality concentrated internally."

Reading the text

Some editing of the translated portion of this text needs explanation. Because terms like t'ai chi ch'uan, ch'i, yin-yang, kung fu, ch'i kung, shaolin boxing and tan t'ien are quite common phrases in books such as this, I do not italicize or explain them within the footnotes of the text. Most were also defined in the first volume of this series.

Chin is always termed as either energy or energies. *Fa* is herein always termed as issue, issued or issuing. Other terms like *t'ui shou* (pushing hands), *san shou* (dispersing hands) and *ta lu* (great roll-back), *ch'uan* (boxing), *sung* (sensitive response/relax), *shen* (spirit), *wei lu* (tail bone region) and all posture names of t'ai chi ch'uan, if used as purely a posture name and not as an energy, are all italicized. These are italicized to draw further attention to them, as they are not commonly used in related materials.

All romanizations of Chinese characters are taken from the Wade-Giles system, not the modern form of *pin-yin*. All brackets are the translator's. All parentheses belong to the original Chinese text, unless I have included a romanization of a character after its Chinese equivalent. All quotes from the classics are mine, most of which can be found in my book *Imagination Becomes Reality*.

All footnotes at the end of each section are the translator's, not part of Chen Kung's original Chinese text. The character for each particular energy being discussed is immediately followed in the footnotes with an etymological definition. Knowing the primitive meaning and derivations can be very helpful in understanding the language of t'ai chi ch'uan. Language, as we all know, can be very misleading, especially when dealing with translations.

In addition to Chen Kung's introduction and the explanation of the energies, I have also included at the end two other pieces from his work, titled, *An Explanation of Restraining, Seizing, Grasping and Closing,* and, *The Principles and Essential Roots of T'ai Chi Ch'uan,* as they are very much related to the subject of energy.

Conclusion

After many years of stop and go, "mugging and bugging," practicing and studying, I can now with a glad heart say, read and enjoy.

Season of Grain Fills
June, 1994
Stuart Alve Olson

The Intrinsic Energies
of T'ai Chi Ch'uan

Volume Two, Chen Kung Series

The Intrinsic Energies Of
T'ai Chi Ch'uan

From *T'ai Chi Ch'uan Tao Chien Kan San-Shou Ho Lun*

By Chen Kung

Translated by Stuart Alve Olson
© 1994

Discourse on Intrinsic Energy

Lun Chin

Introduction

*T*hose without training in the *ch'uan*[1] arts will be incapable of making a clear distinction between external muscular force (*li*) and intrinsic energy (*chin*).[2] Only those with vast knowledge of boxing are capable of clearly analyzing and distinguishing li and chin. Only after many years of practicing and studying martial arts can the differences really be seen, and these can still remain a mystery to some. This is a matter of regret.

We need to absolutely understand that force originates from the bone and from deep within the shoulder blades (scapula), and it is these two areas which prevent energy from being issued. Energy comes from the sinews and can be issued—it can therefore penetrate the four limbs. Force is visible, energy is invisible; force is linear, energy is circular; force is harsh, energy is smooth; force is slow, energy is quick; force is scattered, energy is unified; force floats, energy sinks; force is dull, energy is sharp. In other words, force and energy are not identical.

Shaolin boxing divides force into the *vertical, horizontal, insubstantial* and *substantial*. Vertical force is visible and horizontal force is concealed; insubstantial force is hard and substantial force is soft. Those with little knowledge of *ch'uan* rely on the vertical and insubstantial aspects of force. But those with knowledge rely on the horizontal and substantial aspects of force, as these are related to the energies of t'ai chi ch'uan. However, within these related energies there are further divisions, such as: *cutting, skilled, falling* and *sticking* energies. But again, beginning students rely too much on just the cutting and falling energy.

Cutting energy is too vertical, making it difficult to rise and fall; skilled energy (a limited type of energy) is too inanimate, making it difficult to change and neutralize; falling energy is too hurried, making it too difficult to separate or join. These are forceful types of energy, superficial and not very ingenious. The highest art here has more to do with the skills of sticking energy, which contain the skills of nimbleness and alertness.

When you first attempt the task of issuing energy, it is physically awkward to adapt to being without energy, both before and after striking the opponent. Only by willing it in an instant can the opponent be attacked properly. It must be quick like a flash of lightning or electricity. Once it has been issued it must be immediately withdrawn so that the ch'i can be gathered, the spirit can be retained, and so there will be no expenditure of external muscular force.

Now, yang energy relies on the tensing of the muscles around the bone and yin energy is like a great wind that blows past bending the hundred grasses. In the kung fu of Shaolin boxing, yang energy is the foremost vehicle. In contrast, t'ai chi ch'uan values exclusively the skillful forms of energy, yin energy, and places no value on external muscular force. Those who rely on brute, muscular strength believe the more you emphasize it, the more substantial it becomes. Those favoring skillful energy consider that the more refined the energy, the more expedient its use. Within t'ai chi ch'uan energy has developed into numerous branches, such as:

chan nien (adhering sticking) energy

ting (listening) energy

tung (interpreting) energy

tsou (receiving) energy

hua (neutralizing) energy

chieh (borrowing) energy

fa (issuing) energy

yin (enticing) energy

t'i (raising) energy

chen (sinking) energy

na (seizing) energy

k'ai (opening) energy

ho (closing) energy

po (dispersing) energy

p'eng (ward-off) energy

lu (roll-back) energy

chi (press) energy

an (push) energy

ts'ai (pull) energy

lieh (split) energy

chou (elbow-stroke) energy

kao (shoulder-stroke) energy

ts'o (twisting) energy*

ch'uan (breaking) energy*

chuan (grasping) energy*

tsuan (drilling) energy

chieh (intercepting) energy

leng (frozen) energy*

tuan (interrupting) energy

ts'un (inch) energy*

fen (separating) energy*

tou t'iao (shaky coil) energy*

tou ao (playful shaky) energy*

che tieh (folding up) energy*

ts'a (wiping) energy*

p'i (peeling) energy*

hsu (deceptive) energy*

lin (approaching) energy* ³

So there are these various types of energies within this *ch'uan* art: adhering and sticking , listening , interpreting, and so on. Become well versed and skilled in their special characteristics. When you have truly integrated these energies within yourself, then you will fully appreciate the wonderful mystery of t'ai chi ch'uan.

Although it is said, "T'ai chi ch'uan is the greatest and best of all means for self-cultivation," it is hardly enough to just value mind-intent and not energy. This is because beginning students have to progress step by step. It is through the door that you can enter a house. So you must certainly apply effort in undertaking the development of energy. If you do not understand how to employ energy, then you will also be unclear about the skill of mobilizing the ch'i. If you are unsure about how to employ your ch'i, then the result will be ignorance about the true meaning and relation of mind-intent to t'ai chi ch'uan as well. For it is said, "to reach the top you must begin at the bottom." Also, "to travel far you must begin at the near."

In order to see the true use of energy you must constantly practice the beginning steps and fundamental principles of t'ai chi ch'uan. Therefore, this material

is a compilation of essential points, analyzed and illus-
trated details relating this one specific term, energy, so
that those who are beginning their studies may
research these aspects. For this reason the following
explanation of each energy is given.

Notes:

1. *Ch'uan* is the generic term for boxing and can imply hard as well as soft styles of martial art, such as, Shaolin boxing and t'ai chi ch'uan. The character *ch'uan* depicts a fist within a fist, something hidden and mysterious. Interestingly enough the Chinese, as is revealed in the character *ch'uan*, do not share the West's concept of boxing as an art of strength and speed verses strength and speed. The West places a particular emphasis on strength, and encourages an attitude of aggression. The Chinese concept of boxing is based on skill, calmness of mind and using the opponent's strength against them. Indeed, the English word boxing should most probably not be used as a translation for *ch'uan*. What word should be used is very difficult to determine, so in this text the term *ch'uan* will be retained.

2. *Li* and *chin* (external force as opposed to internal energy). It is these two manners of exhibiting and employing strength that set the hard styles of kung fu apart from the soft styles of the internal arts. Force, in summary, is the process of tightening the muscles around the bone to build strength in the fist, drawing back the arm to build momentum, then initiating the power from the back of the shoulder. The force applied remains yang from inception to completion. Energy (chin), on the other hand, is for the most part, the relaxation of the sinews and tendons around the bone. Initiating the energy from the bottom of the foot, using the whole body as one unit, the energy appears in the hands. This, in analogy, is like the function of a whip. The initial force is applied to the handle of the whip (the foot) and is carried through the length of the whip (legs, waist, spine and arms), yet the whip length is soft and relaxed, not hard and stiff like a stick. The energy is then released

out the tip (the hands) of the whip. Energy is yin in its inception, yang for one instant (while releasing energy) and then immediately yin again (just like a whip). Of course, this is only one aspect of energy. Besides addressing the issuing of energy, sensitivity and the application of both ch'i and spirit will be examined.

3. There are thirty-eight different energies mentioned in this list. However, the explanatory materials to follow discuss only twenty-five. Long energy and lofty towering energy are not mentioned in the above list but are explained in the material. The remaining energies are referred to within the text within the context of another energy, but do not receive their own headings. Those in the above list followed by an asterisk are not given separate headings within the text, but are referred to within the explanation of the other energies.

The Intrinsic Energies

Adhering and Sticking Energy
Chan Nien Chin

铪
黏
勁

Sticking and adhering[1] energy, which cannot easily be discarded[2], acts as an indicator of your progress. Rooted in the *nei chin*[3], it is an absolute requirement in the practice of t'ai chi ch'uan and is developed through *t'ui shou*[4].

When you first train this energy and practice *t'ui shou* your hands are insensitive, like wooden sticks. Gradually, through the repetitious practice of *t'ui-shou*, the hands, arms, chest, spine, and the entire body and skin will become ever more sensitive. Once there is sensitivity, then and only then can you acquire adhering and sticking energy. Then and only then can you make the opponent draw in his breath and resist[5], which will put you in control.

It takes a qualified teacher to demonstrate this adhering and sticking energy, as it is like electricity passing through a battery. The teacher is like someone with electricity who is able to issue an electrical current; the student is like a battery without an electrical charge. Having a teacher demonstrate this is like having electricity pass through your body. A successful demonstration resembles the discharge of electrical energy, as though electricity were being drawn from a battery. The prerequisite is then both a battery and the personal ability to release that electrical energy.

Ordinarily this energy is referred to as "nourishing energy," being like a mother feeding her young children. After awhile the small child learns how to live and eat on their own. When practicing this energy the goal is to reach the highest level. The surface of the skin should become somewhat cloudy in appearance, like a mist or vapor of ch'i, resembling lacquer and glue. Then when your hands come into contact with an opponent your skill will be such that the hands cannot be easily discarded or separated from. Not only the two hands, but the entire body will be like this.

This skill develops your abilities ever higher. The ch'i becomes more substantial and its accumulation even greater. The ch'i will be invisible to the naked eye, but apparent enough for you to definitely sense it. If you then need to use your ch'i with someone of equal skill, you will then also be capable of sensing their level of ch'i.

Once you attach hands in *t'ui shou*, a highly skilled practitioner can immediately know the opponent's level of skill. When adhering and sticking pay close attention to the opponent's circular movements whether large or small. In t'ai chi ch'uan this energy is the most important for *t'ui shou* practice. The first step is obviously to practice. Without practice you will not be able to access any of the other energies. You cannot ignore this beginning practice.

Notes:

1. *Chan* means 'to moisten' and also 'to receive'. The radicals within the character (*shui* for water and *pu*, to seize) render an image of trying to seize water by grasping it. So we have the idea of adherence, like water on the hand.

Nien means 'glutinous', 'a paste' and 'tenacious'. The radicals that make up this character are: *shui* for water, *jen* for man, *ho* for growing crops and *pu*, to seize. So we have the idea of trying to seize something within the wet and muddy fields, from which we derive the meaning of stickiness.

In the commentary section of the *Song of Pushing-Hands* it says to, "adhere, join, stick to and follow ..." At first glance each of these words seems so similar, but in reality each has its own meaning and function within *t'ui shou*. For example, *adhere* means that the opponent can be raised upwards and thus be uprooted; *join* means to "forget yourself and follow the other" so there will be no resistance; *stick to* means to have no separation from the opponent so that you may interpret his movement and intent; *follow* means to adapt and change to the conditions and situation, so that a good opportunity may be created.

In another, more obscure text, *Essential Meanings of the Five Activities*, the energies of adhere and sticking are associated, respectively, with *metal* and *water* of the Five Activities. This correlation extends to *advance step* and *look left* of the thirteen postures of t'ai chi ch'uan.

There are three primary levels of adhering and sticking energy: lower, middle and higher. The lower level involves the ideas of borrowing (*chieh*) energy and enticing (*yin*) energy. This level only requires that you can touch the opponent in order to knock him down with receive (*tsou*) and issue. The middle level involves either the opponent's palm just touching your clothing or your just touching his clothing—at this point he can be knocked down in any of eighteen ways. The highest level of adhering and sticking is where you can pick up and move large or small objects with just the use of an open palm. Such as in the account of Chen Hsiu-feng (Yang Lu-chan's senior disciple) who supposedly lifted an armchair weighing several tens of pounds in order to show Lu-chan's sons, Pan-hou and Chien-hou, that their art was still lacking.

2. The Chinese term *pu tiu*, literally means "can't get rid of," "unable to reject" or "cannot let go of." It is usually translated as "not being able to let go," but I prefer the term *cannot be easily discarded* as it retains the idea of "not being able get rid of" better than just "not letting go". This term should not be confused with *chan nien* (adhere and stick). *Pu tiu* (cannot be easily discarded) is a term specifically meant to describe what the opponent senses when stick and adhere energy is applied to them.

3. *Nei chin* is a generic term, referring to all forms of energies, *ching* (regenerative essence), *ch'i* (breath and vital energy) and *shen* (spirit and mind-intent).

4. The Yang family historical records relate a story about Yang Chien-hou, the second son of Yang Lu-chan (founder of the Yang style system of t'ai chi ch'uan). This story tells how Chien-hou could hold a sparrow in the palm of his hand and make it impossible for the bird to fly away. This was supposedly possible because of Chien-hou's high skill with interpreting energy. As soon as the bird sunk its weight downward to take off, Chien-hou would hollow his palm and hence not give the bird any foothold to push off from his hand. I do not know if this story is true. Having

never seen anyone do this, it is difficult to vouch for its authenticity. However, in theory it is plausible because a bird does need to push off on something in order to begin flight.

Now within t'ai chi ch'uan terminology the compound *t'ui shou* is used to describe "pushing-hands". The character *t'ui* is made up of two radicals, on the left is the main radical of *shou*, which depicts the idea of a hand. On the right is *chui*, which is the symbol for bird. Together they render the idea of 'a bird in the hand'. In everyday Chinese the character *t'ui* retains the multiple meanings of 'to push', 'to yield', 'to hand over' and 'to examine'. So we can see how the story of Chien-hou and the bird coincide with the term *t'ui shou*. Which came first the term, or the story? An older term for pushing hands was *ta shou*. *Ta* means to strike and *shou*, hand. For example, the t'ai chi ch'uan classical work titled, *Ta Shou Ko* (Song of Pushing Hands).

The story does provide a clearer insight into the whole concept of *t'ui shou* practice. The translation of *t'ui shou* might better be rendered as "sensing hands", as the whole idea of keeping a bird in the palm would be the result of sensitivity, not pushing. Pushing in the English language carries the ideas of force and exertion, and there can be none of that if the bird is to remain in the palm. Therefore, in practicing *t'ui shou*, we should apply the language of sensing, not pushing. If we use the English interpretation of 'push', it is easier for the defects of force and exertion to creep into our practice of *t'ui shou*.

5. Getting an opponent to inhale is how to make him substantial and is a technique of adhering, uprooting him by first bringing his breath upwards. Issuing energy to attack at the time of the opponent's inhale will not only create better conditions for your issue, but hinders his ability to neutralize as well.

Listening Energy
Ting Chin

聽
勁

*L*istening[1] is like hearing with your whole skin, a heightened tactile sensitivity. [2] You listen, without using your ears. Before you train in listening energy, you must first train adhering and sticking energy. If you do not understand adhering and sticking energy, you will be unable to listen. *T'ui shou* is the main discipline for developing listening and its perfection leads to interpreting energy. If you are caught unawares, and have no listening skill, you will be unable to interpret, which is the next stage of the process. It would be like engaging in a conversation without using your ears, or listening to silence. Without this energy you will not acquire the skill of apprehending your opponent's intent. You can never hope to interpret without listening.

To develop listening energy in accordance with

t'ai chi ch'uan principle you must first rid yourself of the hindrances of external muscular force. Loosen and relax[3] the waist and legs; meditate on stilling the mind; accumulate the ch'i and concentrate the spirit, otherwise you cannot develop listening.

Without listening, how can you interpret? Without interpreting, how can you receive? Without receiving, how can you neutralize? If there is no neutralize, how can you issue? From this it should be evident that the t'ai chi ch'uan energy of listening is extremely important. Few pay attention to this profound and abstruse practice.

Notes:

1.*Ting* means to hear, listen and understand. The radicals within the character are: (right side, from above) *shih* for complete; *wang* for a net; *i* for one; and *hsin* for mind. On the left side is the radical for the ears, *erh*. Hence, the idea of capturing (understanding) everything (net-like) with a oneness of mind through the use of hearing, listening and comprehending.

The manner in which you develop and learn listening energy is expressed in the *T'ai Chi Ch'uan Classic*, "through silent remembering and thorough examination, you will gradually arrive at the state of being able to follow your own mind. The fundamental here is to forget yourself and follow others." This means "learning how to lose" and "abiding by the tan t'ien," which are the results of forgetting yourself and following others. For in this way you can listen, otherwise your mind is so full of tension and anxiety about protecting yourself and defeating the opponent, that you cannot hear anything else. This is very similar to the Zen adage about coming to the master asking for tea to be poured into your cup, totally unaware that the cup is full in the first place.

Listening is no different, as we are normally unaware that we are so busy listening to ourselves that the opponent cannot be heard. It is extremely important, indeed imperative, that listening energy be acquired, as it is like a bridge connecting the skills of adhering and sticking energy to interpreting energy. To be without interpreting energy means that you must still rely on external muscular force to a great extent. But with interpreting energy, as the *T'ai Chi Ch'uan Classic* states, "you will reach a state of *shen ming*."

2. The listening that is being discussed here is not with the

ear, but rather through the sense of touch. Learning how to touch with a light sensitivity, developed from adhering and sticking energy, you can begin sensing the actions of an opponent. This is like hearing from your fingertips. Eventually your whole skin can listen and sense when touching or being touched. However, if you use tension when touching the opponent all the ability of sensing or listening is destroyed.

3. *Sung* is probably one of the most important terms in t'ai chi ch'uan, yet it is without question the most neglected and misinterpreted concept of the internal arts. *Sung* is normally translated as 'to relax'. But in English the meaning of relax has too much of the idea of 'collapse'. *Sung* on the contrary implies a very high level of alertness, sensitivity, nimbleness and lightness, with an inordinate mindfulness for the conservation of energy.

A cat is the best example of *sung*. We have all seen a cat sleeping (which is more like conserving energy than sleep for the most part), yet if a mouse were to pass by the cat would immediately leap on it. The cat was seemingly in a deep sleep, yet it is so very alert. The cat can also jump ten times its own body height, in part because it can relax (*sung*) all its muscles and bones (lightness and nimbleness), and then in one instant tense them, but then immediately let go again. In t'ai chi ch'uan this is called 'becoming yin to release the yang, returning to yin'. And of course the cat also uses mind-intent (*i*) quite well. Just watch the cat's eyes before it jumps—it's as if the eyes took the mind beforehand to where it will jump.

Again, if we were to watch a cat catching a rat, we would see a lot of good t'ai chi ch'uan at work. First of all upon seeing the rat the cat sinks downwards, lowering its body for a low center of balance. Next, the body of the cat remains still and poised, externally appearing relaxed. Then the eyes become widened and totally focused on the rat (expressing its spirit). The cat lies patiently in wait. If the rat does not move, the cat will not move. The cat is waiting to see the rat's direction of escape and when the rat does try to escape, the cat will head it off at the pass and intercept it.

In contradistinction the dog, when chasing a squirrel, becomes very excited and will run after the squirrel in a straight line. He will run to the spot where the squirrel was originally and then change course mid stream. Confusion and excitement rule the dog, who uses a lot of external muscular force and very little mind-intent.

Sung involves much more than just the idea of relaxation, but equally as well the ideas of sensitivity, alertness, etc. Indeed, many reputable t'ai chi ch'uan texts refer to *sung* as an energy of itself, equal to any mentioned in this work. The reason it is not given its own heading here, is that *sung* is the very *modus operandi* of all energies in t'ai chi ch'uan.

Interpreting Energy
Tung Chin

懂
勁

When you are capable of listening you will then be able to interpret.[1] Pay full and absolute attention, otherwise your listening may be incorrect and the ability to interpret will be incomplete. Interpreting is the first gate, and is also very difficult. Without oral instruction from a reputable teacher you cannot hope to understand it.[2] Only by passing through an appropriate period of practicing t'ai chi ch'uan and *t'ui shou* can you expect to fully understand the methods and principles of this energy.

Before acquiring the skills of interpreting energy it is easy to commit the errors of *opposing, leaning, discarding* and *resisting*. Later, when more accomplished with interpreting energy you will still occasionally commit the errors of *severance, splice, bending down-*

wards and *looking upwards*.[3] Later however this will all improve and it will be like interpreting without having to interpret. The goal is to be completely free from the errors of severance and splice. Which you can readily see would corrupt your listening energy and would prevent you from penetrating the utmost limits of interpreting energy.

When you can naturally move through initiation of mind-intent to *evade, return, attach, clear, circle, change, advance* and *withdraw*[4], then and only then can it be called genuine interpreting energy. After acquiring genuine interpreting energy, you will achieve the profound abilities of "bending and stretching" and "movement and stillness". You will be able to effectively *open-close* and *ascend-descend*. The end result of all these is that you will attain the state known as, "entering the realm of the divine."[5]

In the *T'ai Chi Ch'uan Treatise* it says, "After you acquire interpreting energy, the more you practice, the more skill you will obtain." In response to this verse, previous to interpreting energy you must be able to perceive the one foot, then the one inch, the one tenth of an inch and finally even the one ten-thousandth of an inch. But these are only minor skills, nothing more. It is said, "to be able to deal with an opponent at a one foot distance is hard without first acquiring interpreting energy."

It is certain that after acquiring interpreting energy *shen ming* will appear. From the skills of being able to measure the foot, measuring the inch, the tenth of an inch and even measuring the ten-thousandth of an inch, you will be able to measure everything. Afterwards you will obtain the skills of *restraining, grasping, seizing* and *closing*.[6] You will also be able to distinguish the two types of interpreting energy—your own and your opponent's. Interpreting your own energy is to meet with the divine. This is the *yin* within, where you discover and eliminate the aggression to which we are all so prone.

A common saying states, "The yang attains the yin, water and fire become equal, and *ch'ien* and *k'un* blend to become mercury.[7] This is to nurture the divine within yourself." This is also the central most important secret of attaining the *Tao*.

When interpreting an opponent's energy, listen first, then follow and adapt to all the changes. Do not be over anxious about your posturing and take care not to be entirely motionless.[8]

Attaining this profound skill of interpreting is a most important fundamental in t'ai chi ch'uan. Interpreting your own and your opponent's energy is considered the great achievement of t'ai chi ch'uan. Those who practice t'ai chi ch'uan without interpreting energy do not understand this teaching. Consequently, it is difficult for them to progress in t'ai chi ch'uan.

Notes:

1. The character *tung* is comprised of the main radical *hsin*, meaning heart/mind. On the top, right side, is the radical *tsao*, which means grass, but also carries the meaning of "the origin of things". Underneath *tsao* is the character *chung*, which expresses the idea of important and weighty concerns. The entire character *tung* here represents the ideas of understanding and comprehending, which from the radicals is the image of the mind/heart interpreting the importance of the origin of something. In this case, what is important is to comprehend the inception of an opponent's actions.

   In the *T'ai Chi Ch'uan Classic* it says, "Through self-mastery you will gradually apprehend interpreting energy. From interpreting energy you will reach a state of shen ming (spiritual illumination). But without a long period of arduous practice, you will be unable to suddenly possess a clear understanding." Self-mastery is referring to the solo postures of t'ai chi ch'uan and interpreting energy refers to the two-person exercises. Without first mastering the postures of the solo form you will not have the necessary foundation for acquiring interpreting energy, such as root, relaxation, ch'i accumulation and mobilization, and the abilities associated with the spirit and mind-intent. If you cannot sense these things in your own body and self, how can you ever expect to do so with an opponent? Interpreting energy is the skill of comprehending an opponent's root (center of balance), substantial and insubstantial (the quality of their *sung*), the breath (ch'i), alertness (state of their *shen*) and their intent. Again, the *T'ai Chi Ch'uan Classic* states, "The opponent does not know me, but I alone know him." You know him because you know yourself; to know yourself is to know others.

2. This line comes directly from the *Song of Substance and Function of the Thirteen Postures*. Interpreting is to a great extent tactile so to experience the sensation, to feel it demonstrated on you yourself is invaluable. It wouldn't benefit you much for a teacher to only talk about these skills and never demonstrate them. The teacher must be able to show you so that you can understand and experience for yourself, otherwise your learning will be limited and in vain.

3. These eight defects or errors (*opposing, leaning, discarding, resisting, severance, splice, bending downwards* and *looking upwards*) are the negative aspects of the Eight Postures (*ward-off, roll-back, press, push, pull, split, elbow-stroke* and *shoulder-stroke*). When these eight defects are eliminated then interpreting is second nature and you won't have to concern yourself with the idea that you are interpreting. Thus we have the idea in the next line, "interpreting without having to interpret."

4. These are the positive aspects of the Eight Postures (*evading, returning, attaching, clearing, circling, changing, advancing* and *withdrawing*). It is these which constitute the genuine skill of interpreting energy.

5. *Shen ming* in common Chinese usage means the 'Gods', but not in the Christian sense of the word, more like that of the gods in Greek mythology. However, in Taoism the term *shen ming* refers to a state of mind which is god-like, which is to be spiritually illumined, such as in the case of immortals. But certain levels of immortality are considered spiritually higher than that of even gods. In t'ai chi ch'uan the term in one sense carries exactly the same meaning as in Taoism, but it also implies a state of mind which is extreme-

ly perceptive of conditions. Therefore, within t'ai chi ch'uan *shen ming* means something closer to "clear mind" or "spiritual clarity".

6. A more detailed explanation follows in the last section of this book, under the heading of *An Explanation of Restraining, Seizing, Grasping and Closing*. Briefly, *chieh* means "restraining the vessels"; *na*, "seizing the meridians"; *chua*, "grasping the sinews"; and, *pi* means "closing the cavities".

7. These Taoist verses reveal much about the internal aspects of interpreting energy. In brief, *the yang attaining its yin* is in one sense conveying the idea that the body and mind have reached a state of tranquillity and harmony. But in reference to t'ai chi ch'uan, this is a statement about the balance of yin and yang. For the underlying function of t'ai chi ch'uan is in the distinguishing of substantial (yang) and insubstantial (yin). Total reliance on strength is yang; total reliance on energy is yin. Hence, when strength becomes or reaches the state of energy, interpreting energy is then a kinetic function.

   Water represents the blood and fire represents, the ch'i. When the ch'i, which is like a latent oxygen, integrates fully with the blood, then there is "free circulation" of ch'i throughout the body. When ch'i flows freely throughout the body, your sensitivity and awareness are greatly heightened, hence the interpreting energy is developed.

   Ch'ien and *k'un* are terms from the *I-Ching* (Book of Changes). *Ch'ien* represents heaven and pure yang; *k'un*, earth and pure yin. *Mercury* is a Taoist metaphor for 'elixir', i.e., elixir of immortality and is sometimes referred to as "cinnabar". So the blending or mixing of yin and yang is the elixir. Again, achieving this level, called "attaining the

Tao" would create the conditions of interpreting energy skills, without question.

8. The text has now returned to a more practical discussion of interpreting energy. In learning to interpret you should never attempt to be in a hurry and so become anxious. The mental tension alone will obstruct your ability to interpret. Likewise, you can't sit motionless like a piece of wood either. For these reason the text instructs that you should "listen" (feel, sense, let go, etc.) and adapt to all the changes the opponent makes—"adhere, join, stick to and follow, and don't resist"—just be in accord with the opponent. Interpreting is then a natural occurrence. Don't try to either force it, nor become inattentive. Be like the cat watching the rat, then you can interpret.

Receiving Energy
Tsou Chin

*R*eceiving[1] is the energy of "not-going-against."[2] Its principal method involves "drawing back."[3] Receiving energy derives from interpreting energy. How could you receive if you could not first interpret? An opponent may attack, high or low, from the side or straight ahead, from the left or right, or from a long or a short distance. So to achieve the highest level of receiving energy you cannot have a fixed plan of action.[4] If you cannot interpret his strength, how could you hope to receive it?

Receiving means to receive and destroy the opponent's sense of balance and strength, without giving him any sense of resistance when you come together. When doing *t'ui shou* the palms of the hands must immediately sense the intent and center of balance of the opponent, then just as immediately change to emptiness. If you go out to meet your opponent and place your weight on him, you must relax,[5] or if you go out to meet him double-weighted[6] then you must sink.[7] In order to drain away his strength follow the direction of the opponent's energy and then get rid of it, without the slightest resistance. Wherever he moves the opponent will meet with nothing. But you must not use strength! That is to say, "If the left is weighted, then the left becomes insubstantial; if the right is weighted, then the right should disappear."

When first learning this energy students do not want to go out and meet with a great energy to receive it. This means they have the mind-intent of resistance.[8] True receiving will later need no interpreting energy. The very axis of receiving energy lies entirely in the waist and legs. If the waist and legs are without skill then it will all be in vain. You must practice receiving energy so as not to be caught unawares.

Notes:

1. *Tsou* literally means "to walk," which leads to the idea of "going to." A good analogy for receiving energy is that of a soccer goalie. Seeing the ball coming the goalie will step out to lightly touch the ball with his hands. This softens the incoming force and gives him better control over the ball as he draws it back into himself. To just stand there and deflect the ball will result in losing control over the ball. So in t'ai chi ch'uan first receive an incoming force to both better control it and to deaden its energy.

The *T'a'i Chi Ch'uan Classic* states, "To adhere is to receive; to receive is to adhere." The moment you attach to the opponent you are in essence receiving, but only if you are drawing in his strength. Take about seventy percent of his incoming force, bringing it down through your rear leg into the foot so that it may be issued back to him. This is just one way of receiving, but no matter the method, you must be able to adhere properly otherwise receiving will be of no use.

2. *Pu ting* (not-going-against) is expressing the idea that you should never view receiving as pitting strength against strength, resisting the incoming force. That is certainly not the idea of going out to receive an incoming attack.

3. *Hou tui* (drawing back) means to attach lightly, without resistance, and then draw your body and the incoming energy back. Again, this is like the soccer goalie, who softens the blow of the incoming ball by leading it in.

4. To *have a fixed plan of action* has two important meanings. The *first* has to do with what is referred to in every other style of martial art, "a fighting stance." T'ai chi ch'uan has

no fixed fighting stance. Standing upright, in a relaxed and casual manner, is as close to a fighting stance as t'ai chi ch'uan gets. To appear open and vulnerable, not closed and impregnable, is what t'ai chi ch'uan refers to as "open the door to let the robber in." To be closed and appearing impregnable only reveals to the opponent what their course of action should be; they can see what is open and what is closed; the strong points and defects; the substantial and insubstantial aspects of your body, and most importantly, what style of martial art you are using. Conversely, to be standing relaxed and open gives no indication of anything threatening or requiring any strategy on the opponent's part. However, what this affords you is the ability to not only interpret, but receive the in-coming actions of the opponent. But to accomplish these your mind and body must be relaxed and calm. Tension, anxiety and fixed thinking will only get you defeated.

Secondly. Before the opponent attacks, you cannot tell yourself that you will use, say, *brush left knee and twist step* , to counter his attack. This, again, is *a fixed plan of action* and only limits you, just as a fixed fighting stance does. The reaction to an attack must be spontaneous, let the spirit, energy and ch'i come out naturally. Once you adhere to an opponent, your technique will come out according to the circumstance. This is like the analogy, water flows not by plan, but by naturally entering the low places. Many will find difficulty in this, but those who do are also those who have not practiced genuinely the training exercises of *t'ui shou, san shou* and *ta lu,* and more so have not studied the t'ai chi ch'uan classics in any detail. Many t'ai chi*ists,* who cannot accomplish this level, usually incorporate kung fu techniques to compensate and so end up relying on fixed plans of action.

In conclusion, *The Mental Elucidation of the Thirteen*

Kinetic Postures, says: "When standing, the body must be centered, upright and comfortable, and able to sustain an attack from any of the eight directions."

5. See note 3 under *Listening Energy*.

6. *Shuang chung* (double weightedness) is one of the most common errors and misunderstood principles of t'ai chi ch'uan practitioners. In the *T'ai Chi Ch'uan Classic* attributed to Wang Chung-yueh it states, "*Sinking the weight to one side results in adapting to circumstances. Double weightedness results in being impeded. Often we see those who after many years of painstaking effort cannot employ a neutralization and are generally subdued by an opponent. This is because they have not understood the fault of double weighting. In wanting to avoid this fault you must know yin and yang.*"

First of all, double weightedness *does not* mean that there is equal weight on both feet. Many t'ai chi ch'uan forms call for stances with weight percentage distributions of sixty-forty, seventy-thirty, eighty-twenty—one leg receiving more weight than the other. However, the defect of double weightedness has nothing to do with discerning those percentages. It has everything to do with sinking the majority of your weight into one leg or another during movement. Double weightedness applies to three situations: 1) the body must be in motion to commit the error of double weighting, as it does not apply to standing postures; 2) being able to clearly discriminate the substantial (yang) from the insubstantial (yin) of each part of your body, not just the legs. Meaning, in part, that when an opponent pushes on your body you will be able to change your center of balance without resistance or getting trapped into one leg or the other, and; 3) not letting one side of the body become purely substantial. Meaning that double weightedness is created when you are, for example, pushing off your front right leg and simultaneously pushing with your right hand (if the opponent grabs your right hand you can be pulled off your front leg and your energy can be extended off your center), or when an opponent pushes on your right side and you sink into the right leg (if the opponent then immediately removes his pushing hand you will fall forward off your center). Another defect which relates to this is called *double floating* and this is caused by pushing, for example, with both legs rising upwards simultaneously with no sinking applied into the opposite leg of the push.

7. *Sinking*, see *Sinking Energy*.

8. The mind-intent of resistance comes from self-protection. T'ai chi ch'uan in application is "in-fighting", for lack of a better term. The whole idea of t'ai chi ch'uan is to take away an opponent's center. If they have no center, they cannot stand up. But initially there is a fear of being right next to an opponent to take away their center, and when you are next to the opponent there is then a resistance and struggle against any movement by the opponent. Rather, you should learn to apply "learning how to lose", "investing in loss" and "abiding by the *tan t'ien*." All these are related and have to do with learning the error and defect of resistance. For nothing confuses and disrupts an opponent's actions more than having someone go to them (receiving) when they strike out; having to attack someone who is relaxed during the attack, and; finding nothing to grab onto or strike against (insubstantial and without the defect of double weightedness).

Neutralizing Energy
Hua Chin

化勁

Neutralizing[1] energy comes from sticking energy and receiving energy, yet is also complete within itself. It 'cannot be easily discarded' and is a 'non-resistant' energy. You can neutralize the opponent by following in accord with their movements. *Advance, withdraw, look left* and *gaze right*[2] mutually support each other and are not separate activities. The important point with neutralizing energy is to follow the opponent completely until you can turn his back towards you. Your opponent may have the strength of over a thousand catties, but it will be of no use to him if you can achieve this skill. So neutralizing energy is truly very important within t'ai chi ch'uan. Within this neutralizing energy a little ward-off (*p'eng*) energy[3] must exist. Without ward-off energy you will be unable to neutralize. With neutralizing energy it is important not to make use of the hands or shoulders; use the waist and legs entirely. Using the hands and shoulders is called 'stiff removal'[4] and is not the true neutralizing energy of t'ai chi ch'uan.

If possible follow the opponent's movement, whether it be high or low, to the side or straight ahead, and fast or slow movements. (If the neutralization is too hurried, you will be unable to entice him into the point of a funnel.[5] The error in being too slow is that there is no neutralization or removal). Adhere and then neutralize.

Depending on whether the neutralization results from a crooked or straight movement, from the right or left, or from above or below you need to change the direction [6] of the opponent's line of energy. In application always pay attention and adapt to circumstances. So when moving "to and fro" keep the intent of folding-up; advance and withdraw must have the intent of circular-change[7], causing the opponent to be totally unaware of your line of energy. Always direct his energy to the side, causing his back to turn and then stop at this point. This is called true neutralizing energy.

After having neutralized you can seize or issue,[8] but do not exhaust the neutralization. If the neutralization is taken to the point of exhaustion this will make it easy to sever the adhering and sticking energy and your power will then be lost and your following separated. Afterwards you will be unable to neutralize. Your back will be turned to the opponent and you will be incapable of advancing.

To neutralize an opponent's issued energy you must move when the opponent's energy is just about to be released. As it begins to be issue, follow the energy and neutralize it without being too early [hurried] or too late [slow]. If you are too early and nothing has come to you, then there is no neutralization. If you are too late then your neutralization will be of no advantage to you.

Neutralization may employ big or small circles. The very highly skilled use very small circles, the lesser skilled use big circles. Some consider t'ai chi ch'uan to be just an accentuation of yielding and neutralizing. This is entirely wrong. In genuine *ch'uan* there is both neutralizing and issuing. Through neutralization, power is acquired, which develops issuing and other natural abilities. If this power is not acquired through neutralizing, how can you issue? This comes entirely from practicing and understanding the applications.

The highly skilled can advance after neutralizing. The body moves back to neutralize and withdraw, but at the same time there is an advancing without stepping forward. This is regarded as the method of withdrawing to perform advance—which is truly mysterious and inconceivable.

On the other hand, the greater portion of beginning students, consider that after neutralizing there is withdraw step. They are unaware that this is just running away and not true neutralizing.

The highly skilled are externally very yielding and soft; internally very unyielding and strong. This strength comes from not having the mind-intent of strength. If you practice daily like this, with effort, you will certainly augment your internal energy. But the difficulty here is to internally embody strength and yet not exhibit it externally. Then when neutralizing an opponent, use yielding and softness to overcome the unyielding and strong. Make use of the opponent's strength and exhaust it through neutralizing until nothing is left.

How mysterious and abstruse are the steps of this kung fu. Requiring no adhering, sticking, joining or following, because you have acquired the skills of interpreting energy, you have penetrated the conditions of *shen ming*.[8] But if you are unable to penetrate the mystery of lightness and nimbleness then you will have trouble easily "removing a thousand catties with four ounces."

Notes:

1. *Hua* (neutralize) contains two radicals. The one on the left, *jen*, represents man or person; *pi* on the right means a spoon or ladle. The character *hua* translates as transformation. In Taoism the more ancient and technical version of *hua* depicts an alchemist stirring the elixir with his ladle. This conveys both the idea of transformation and the process of teaching others, to bring about change and conversion. *Pi* by itself in ancient China also meant to die, but combined with *jen* came to mean the evolution of a flower, transformation, a kind of repetitive rebirth process abetted by human effort.

Later *hua* developed in its meaning from transformation to change, from change to conversion, from conversion to the idea of overthrowing, and now in t'ai chi ch'uan language, to neutralize. I would suspect the term neutralize is used here because of the connotation of "change and overthrow." To neutralize means changing not only the direction of an opponent's attack, but also diffusing and destroying his energy (overthrow), and finally to take that energy and use it against him (transform). In *The Mental Elucidation of the Thirteen Kinetic Postures Treatise* it says, *"to withdraw [neutralize] is to attack; to attack is to withdraw."* In t'ai chi ch'uan your neutralize *is* an attack; you must give back what the opponent gave you. For example, in the story about the reputed founder of t'ai chi ch'uan, a Sung dynasty Taoist monk, Chang San-feng, invented t'ai chi ch'uan after watching a magpie attacking a snake. In brief, when the magpie struck the head of the snake, the snake's tail struck the bird; when the bird struck the tail, the snake's head attacked, and when the bird attacked the middle of the snake, both the tail and head attacked. From this developed the ideas of "folding up", "neutralize-attack" and "receive-attack" in t'ai chi ch'uan. Hence, with folding up, if someone pushes on your wrist, the elbow folds and attacks; pushing on your elbow, the shoulder attacks; pushing on the shoulder, the head attacks.

In regards to *neutralize-attack*, if someone attacks and puts weight on your left side, the right side attacks. *Receive-attack* means to draw in about seventy percent of the opponent's incoming force by redirecting it into your rooted leg and then, like a metal spring pushed down, you rise instantly off that leg to repel the opponent back. There are of course numerous other examples of each technique which could be provided here, but these should suffice to make the idea clear. When examining the idea of *hua*, as neutralize, it is easy to see that an opponent's energy is always being transformed, changed and converted right back into himself. It is for these reasons that the text clearly states, "neutralizing energy comes from adhering and receiving energy."

2. *Advance step, withdraw step, look left, gaze right,* and along with *central equilibrium* make up what is called the Five Activities, which represent five of the thirteen postures of t'ai chi ch'uan. The other eight being the eight postures of *ward-off, roll-back, press, push, pull, split, elbow-stroke* and *shoulder-stroke.*

The text states that *advance, withdraw, look left* and *gaze right* are not completely separate activities. That is to say, there is no advance without the intent to withdraw, and vice versa; no look left without the intent to gaze right, and vice versa; when withdrawing there must always be the intent to either look left or gaze right, and vice versa; when advancing there must be the intent of either look left or gaze right. In other words, no matter what the situation you must be able to adapt to all the opponent's changes. If

the opponent advances, you withdraw, but advance immediately when his energy is neutralized. The techniques of
"folding up", "neutralize-attack" and "receive-attack"
reflect four of the five activities. Central equilibrium is an
aspect of all previous four activities and eight postures.

3. When neutralizing there must always be the hidden
intention of ward-off energy, otherwise the psychology is
only to neutralize. If the opponent senses your neutralization and changes you will be caught unawares. Another
manner of viewing this lies in the t'ai chi ch'uan usage of
reverse-psychology. *When being pushed, act as if you were
pulling the opponent in; when pushing, act as if the opponent
pulled you in.* This idea solves many problems for the practitioner of *t'ui shou.* 1) It takes away the tension of resistance
in the arms. 2) It allows for more control over the opponent.
3) You can apply the energies of adhering and sticking,
receiving and interpreting with much greater sensitivity
and awareness. 4) The opponent cannot comprehend your
intentions. 5) The applications of the five essentials of
adhere, join, stick to, follow, and do not let go-do not resist are
more readily understood and applied. In conclusion,
pulling the opponent in is to have the intent of ward-off
energy because the opponent can be repelled immediately
at anytime during the neutralizing if he changes his intention.

4. This simply means that the arms and hands try to muscle
the opponent into a defective position, but this will not
work, you must use the waist and legs. In the *T'ai Chi
Ch'uan Treatise* it says, "*Failure to obtain a superior position
and create a good opportunity results from the body being in a
state of disorder and confusion. To correct this fault adjust the
waist and legs.*" Note that the text does not say, "adjust the

hands and arms." The hands and arms remain relaxed and adhere to the opponent, ready to be the expression of energy, that is to issue energy.

5. The idea of enticing energy is precisely this, drawing an opponent into a point of no return, like water flowing into the apex of a cone or funnel.

6. *Fang hsiang* means the direction or course that the opponent's energy is going to.

7. See note 2, this section. "To and fro" is related to *look left* and *gaze right*, and thus folding up techniques are to be applied; advancing and withdrawing are *advance step* and *withdraw step*, and the techniques of circular-change, i.e., neutralize-attack and receive-attack are to be applied.

8. Neutralize (*hua*), seize (*na*) and attack (*fa*). These three energies comprise the entire basis of t'ai chi ch'uan as a means of self-defense. In learning the two-person sets of Yang style t'ai chi ch'uan, there are three divisions of exercises: *san shou* (dispersing hands), *t'ui shou* (sensing hands), and *ta lu* (great roll-back). Within each of these exercises the individual postures/applications are taught so that the student realizes that within each posture and application there are the aspects of neutralize, seize and attack (issue).

Enticing Energy
Yin Chin

引
動

nticing[1] energy is applied when the opponent does not move and you must then entice him to move.[2] If the opponent is in motion, you also must entice him into a correct line. An opponent may know a sufficient amount about neutralizing, seizing and issuing energies, yet not know of enticing energy or know that enticing energy truly occurs between neutralize and seize,[3] with the neutralization being the most difficult.

Suppose that an opponent attacks you and you are unable to follow your own inclinations. In this case you must clearly use enticing energy in order to entice him into a defective position. When two people are walking in opposite directions, there is no way for them to meet with each other. Clearly they have to be induced to meet. The acquisition of enticing skill is similar to this.

You must neutralize the opponent's energy at the time it is just about, but not completely, exhausted. Then and only then do you entice him to come in completely. In other words, enticing energy seeks to lead the opponent into a defective position, to focus on his center.

You will certainly have little difficulty when encountering an opponent with shallow skills. But suppose you meet with someone who does have some abilities. Then you need to make use of the enticing method. Entice above to strike below; entice straight away to attack crosswise, or perhaps you fake an outgoing punch in order to entice him and cause his ch'i to rise upwards from the tan t'ien and make his center of balance unstable. This will cause him to become alarmed and disordered, and he will be caught completely unawares.[4] You can then seize and issue. So before issuing there must be seizing; before seizing there must be enticing; before enticing there must be neutralizing—this is the proper order to be maintained.

The methods of enticing energy are not specialized, but do take years of difficult practice, because enticing energy is not only enticing with the hands, but equally there is the required use of the body, stepping and waist[5] methods.

Now, the longer the enticing is, the more powerful becomes the issuing. Therefore, in the *T'ai Chi Ch'uan Treatise* it says, "When advancing it seems to become ever longer; when withdrawing it seems to become ever closer." This is the intention of enticing. In closing, do not ignore the two concepts of "adhering and sticking", then you will always be paying attention.

Notes:

1. *Yin* means "to draw a bow." From this comes the ideas of enticing, leading, drawing out and inducing. The character *yin* is comprised of two radicals. *Kung*, the main radical on the left, represents a curved bow; *kun* on the right, is the bow string. So by pulling on a bow-string, the arrow in the bow in then guided out, leading to a particular target, much as an opponent is led and enticed, to a particular defective position. In *The Mental Elucidation of the Thirteen Kinetic Postures* it says, "Storing the energy is like drawing a bow; issuing the energy is like shooting an arrow. Seek the straight from the curved; store and then issue." To *seek* is the entice or leading; *straight* refers to the arrow, or the *energy* to be issued; *curved* refers to the bow and bow-string; pulling back on the bow-string refers to *storing*, and; releasing the arrow refers to *issuing*.

2. In *The Mental Elucidation of the Thirteen Kinetic Postures*, it says: "If the opponent does not move, you do not move. At the slightest movement of the opponent, you begin moving." For a very long time the idea of enticing an opponent to move created some controversy in the t'ai chi ch'uan community. This largely originated from literal interpretations, from English translations, of this verse. The text distinguishes here between enticing an opponent who is in motion and an opponent who is stationary. The controversy focuses on the enticement of a stationary opponent. If we examine the character *tung*, we see that its two radicals depict the idea of heaviness (*chung*) and strength (*li*). Originally the meaning of *chung* symbolized an intent to rise off the ground; *li* was the energy and strength put into the task. The idea was to depict man's inherent desire to fly or leave the earth, coupled with a sense of the energy being

too heavy for the task (another way of looking at gravity). But *tung* has since come to mean movement: to excite, to rouse, to take action. The meaning of *tung* carries with it the idea of intent or desire to do. *At the slightest movement...* could also be interpreted as, *at the slightest intent*. Suppose your opponent is holding a gun, pointing directly at you. Do you wait to hear the gun fire before moving, or would you attempt to lead the gun barrel to another direction before it fired? Let me demonstrate this with a story I heard from my teacher, Master Tung-tsai Liang.

Master Liang and his teacher, Prof. Cheng Man-ch'ing, taught in New York city during the early sixties. On one occasion a man came to the studio to check out t'ai chi ch'uan, to see if it could be used for martial art. It turns out that this man was a Golden Glove boxer. He had asked Cheng if it would be okay to have t'ai chi ch'uan demonstrated to him. Cheng agreed and told the man to throw some punches at him. The man threw a volley of punches and jabs at Cheng, but all were just feints. After a number of these, Cheng put out his hands and knocked the man down. After getting up the man was astonished that Cheng knew which particular punch was the real one, meant to knock him out. Cheng told him it was in his eyes.

There are four basic ways or stages in which to interpret an opponent's strike. The *first* is what all who are untrained in the *ch'uan* arts do, to react to the opponent after he has struck you. This is clumsy strength (*li*). *Secondly*, with training we begin seeing when the opponent's hand and arm are just coming out and can neutralize it. This is skillful energy. *Thirdly*, we can perceive the opponent drawing in his energy before striking, because for a punch to be released the corresponding shoulder must first rise; a kick, the opposite shoulder must sink. At this stage you can apply any of the energies and issue. This is interpreting energy. The *fourth* stage is actually a continuation of the third. You can see the intent in the opponent's eyes before he draws in to strike and you can therefore take action before he does. This is the stage of *shen ming*.

3. This can be understood by examining the movements of *t'ui shou*. As the opponent begins pushing on your arm, which is in the ward-off position, you should be leading him back (act as if pulling him into yourself). The movement of going back is the neutralize; leading him back is the enticing, and; turning to do roll back is the seize. The neutralize is more difficult in regards to incorporating entice only if the opponent has some knowledge of neutralize, seize and issue energies.

4. *Causing his ch'i to rise upwards from the tan t'ien, making his center of balance unstable. He will become alarmed and disordered, caught completely unawares.* These two sentences in many ways encapsulate the very essence of internal *ch'uan*. In more practical terms, this is saying that if you fake a punch or push to an opponent, they will do a number of things in order to protect themselves. First the breath will rise up into the lungs, causing the upper body to lean forward. The feet will rise up onto the toes and the toes clutch the ground to retain a foothold. There will be a momentary sense of nothing holding them up and so they then struggle in a panic to get back to their center in order to be stable. Depending upon the amount of energy the opponent puts into his protecting, he can either just teeter a little or even fall down of his own accord. It is at this precise moment that you can entice or issue with the expenditure of very little energy. This entire sequence of events occurred because the breath rose upwards, because the opponent could neither interpret nor sink his ch'i into the tan t'ien. Therefore,

the lesson of t'ai chi ch'uan is in many respects, relearning and training yourself to sink, relax and keep the breath low when being attacked. Just like the cat seeing the rat. Otherwise you will lose your center of balance, become alarmed and disordered, and be caught unawares.

5. This is a reference to the Five Methods, which are: *the hands, the eyes, the body, the technique* and *stepping* methods. Each method contains certain principles for the proper function of each method. For example, the eyes must follow the waist in order for the line of vision to be concentrated; the eyes must not be held too widely open nor should the eyelids be lowered. If too widely opened the spirit will become confused and the ch'i will rise into the head; if the eyelids are lowered the spirit will become weakened and from the dullness created, the ch'i will disperse. The error here is that the waist method is actually within the body method and should not be considered separate.

Seizing Energy
Na Chin

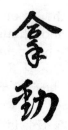

*S*eizing[1] energy is comparable to the two energies of enticing and neutralizing, but is more difficult in practice. It is a very important energy within t'ai chi ch'uan. If you are unable to seize, then you will be incapable of issuing. Yet, if you can seize, then and only then can you issue. If not, issuing will be of no use. The inability to issue stems from incorrect seizing—the vanguard of issuing is seizing.

As soon as you seize, issue without thought, so that you realize your intention and you focus entirely on the issuing. Then you will never miss hitting the mark. Only, when seizing, your movements must be light and nimble. Heaviness will cause the opponent to easily perceive your intentions and so change to neutralize, throwing you off. The opponent will be unable to throw you off if your seizing happens just an instant after your opponent's intention to attack.

This is the subtlety of seizing, subtle in that the opponent is both unaware and unconscious of your intentions. Yet to truly seize an opponent you must seize his moveable joints, such as his wrists, elbows or shoulders.[2] If you do not then it will be easy for you to become the object of neutralize or of severance. Seizing the opponent with both hands should resemble the cross beam of a steelyard scale. Heaviness means, *externally*, your weighting of the scale; lightness means, *internally*, your shifting of the weight. It is essential that you match the high and low sides of the beam with corresponding lightness and heaviness, so that you don't fall off.

When seizing, sink the shoulders and suspending the elbows; hollow the chest and raise the back; also, gather the ch'i, concentrate the spirit, and pay close attention to your center of balance. It is also essential that the *wei lu* be centered and upright; the top of the head suspended, the stance secure and, the center of balance stable and firm. It is commonly said, "when seizing an opponent do not pass over the knee; passing over the knee is not seizing."[3] Going over the knee will cause you to become separated from the opponent and kept at a distance, without your being able to then advance step. If you cannot advance step you will become overly anxious, causing you to lose your center of balance.

Seize an opponent without grasping with the hands; if the hands grasp it will be inefficient and easy to neutralize. The pivotal axis for seizing lies entirely in the waist and legs. You must seize the opponent without forceful grabbing.[4] To just foolishly seize with force makes it very easy for the opponent to get rid of you. It is entirely the mind-intent and ch'i that sets the seize into motion. The stepping methods, body methods and direction of the issue are of equal importance. If this was not mentioned here, the teaching would never be handed down to others.

Those with very abstruse skills are able to seize opponents immediately the hands join, regardless of their actual position. You accomplish seizing the moment you have made the opponent apprehensive. Just by enticing the opponent you will make him susceptible to your seize and cause him to lose all self control and to follow your own intentions.

There is a common saying, "Put them into a funnel."[5] Only the highly skilled can time after time seize, yet never need to issue. Because of this principle you can later seize merely by the laying of the hands. The opponent will know that their strength has been overcome and that they have certainly lost. They recognize that they have unwittingly submitted. There is then no need for you to issue, as the opponent would only experience an unbearable defeat. This is also the *Tao* of the wise man.

Seizing is also divided into two types, visible and invisible. *Visible* means using small circles for seizing. This is a very abstruse kung fu. Big circles, on the other hand, are a very shallow kung fu and easy to comprehend. When two opponents stick together skin to skin and each attempt to entice or seize, their posturing and circles may be easy to comprehend. *Invisible* refers to those who can conceal their circles with a very abstruse level of skill. This type of kung fu is very profound and marvelous. But this energy of invisible seizing can only be acquired through the teachings of a reputable master. Without training myself continually, I would have been unable to achieve success with this energy.

Notes:

1. *Na* is made up of two radicals. *Ho* above means harmony, to join, to shut or close. The lower, main radical, *shou* means the hand(s). As will be seen this character and the above meanings are quite appropriate for this energy.

2. This means to render the joints of the arms, including the joints of the fingers, "dead" or immovable through locking them. This particular form of seizing comes from a separate *ch'uan* art called, *chin na*, "seizing and grappling." This art has been applied to almost every martial art. However, in t'ai chi ch'uan, the actual grappling (*chin*) has been discarded and all seizing is accomplished through circular and binding type actions, rather than actual grasping techniques, which makes use of external muscular force. See note 4 of this section.

3. This is another way of stating the t'ai chi ch'uan principle of *do not let the knee pass over the toes*. When t'ai chi ch'uan was first introduced to the West, many of these principles were erroneously taken in the literal sense. In the Yang style of t'ai chi ch'uan "not letting the knee pass over the toes" refers to a situation when your weight is in the front leg, such as the *bow and arrow* stance. This principle does not apply to the rear leg. The calf should be upright and vertical, so that if you looked down you could see your toes. This is "not letting the knee pass over the toes." Some falsely interpreted this to mean that the knee could bend and extend to the front, as long as the tip of the knee cap did not pass over the tip of the toes. This only serves to put undue pressure on the hip joint, knee and ankle joint. Likewise, it creates the condition of extending your energy, which opponents can take advantage of. This interpretation

caused many doctors to have their doubts about t'ai chi ch'uan, because many t'ai chi*ists* were suffering from chronic strained knee joints.

4. To *forcefully grab* is a true defect in t'ai chi ch'uan. Seizing has more to do with grabbing in a manner similar to how a baby would grab your finger, without forceful tension. Their fingers simply wrap around the finger and adhere. To attempt to use muscular force will only cause the opponent to immediately detect your action and so he can neutralize it. To demonstrate this, have someone grasp your wrist very tightly, and for the moment tighten your wrist and arm muscles to resist his strength. Now try to turn and pull your arm away from his grip. It will prove very difficult. Next, have your partner do the same to your wrist again, only this time you completely relax the muscles in your wrist and arm. Now, simply turn your wrist and pull it out. You will find this to be very easy. For this, and many other reasons, grabbing with force will only serve to be your enemy, as it is your strength which becomes your downfall. Lao Tzu said, *"The tongue lasts a long time because it is soft; the teeth are the first to go because they are hard."*

5. This means that once you touch the opponent he will be trapped, like water poured into a funnel, it has nowhere to go but through the conic section. Once the opponent is in this conic section so to speak, he is defective, meeting with no resistance, losing his center of balance, so forth. Therefore, the text said earlier, "if you can seize, then and only then can you issue," because it creates the conditions for issuing without the use of force.

Issuing Energy
Fa Chin

發勁

Y ou cannot initiate an attack against an opponent without issuing[1] energy. If you have no knowledge of issuing energy, how can you attack an opponent? Much less talk about any other boxing or fighting methods. Those who just practice t'ai chi ch'uan to nourish the body can say nothing about issuing energy. Those who just seek self-defense techniques are likewise ignorant of issuing energy. Because t'ai chi ch'uan practiced like this means you scarcely know how to neutralize and know nothing of issuing. This is knowing how to *guard*, but not knowing how to *attack*.

You must know that within neutralize there are times when the hand-to-hand actions cannot be neutralized. Besides, how can you push and yet do nothing? For once there is defeat and failure, you are then completely compromised. Here are some words of advice, even if you do not wish to overcome the opponent, at least you ought not to be defeated by the opponent.

If there is no neutralization, there can be no issuing (this is a guarding and an attack). Without a neutralization you'll be unable make the opponent extend all his force so you can issue. You must also take into account the neutralization. In the past they would say, "when moving the hands out, you see only red."[2] Once the hand reaches outward the opponent is certainly knocked down.

Never give an opponent an opportunity to guard and attack, or put yourself in the position of having to guard and attack. This way you will avoid many potential threats to your spirit and vitality. These words truly embody principles. If you don't pay full attention to this, then you must pay attention to guarding and attacking, because your spirit and vitality will become divided and dispersed. A person is taken advantage of through the defects of their character.

In t'ai chi ch'uan issuing energy contains the subsets of intercepting, long, sinking, drilling, inch, separating, frozen, interrupting and shaky springing. Among these, intercepting energy is more fierce than long energy; drilling energy is more harsh than sinking energy, and separating energy is more violent than inch energy.

With regard to frozen energy, you must rely on enticing and issuing to the opponent in order to catch him unawares. The power of this energy is extremely fierce, but to make use of this power is certainly not easy. If you do not attain the highest level of this energy, you will be obstructed from attaining the wise man's *Tao*.

What is interrupting energy? Interrupting energy requires that the opponent be enticed so that afterwards you will obtain a good position. With the slightest interruption of the opponent's internal energy, immediately gather up all your energy and then issue directly to the opponent's body. This type of energy is extremely fierce. Even if you do not exactly know how to use this "supreme ultimate" energy, or perhaps you do know it, but it is not very refined, the effectiveness will still be unbelievable. To endure the training is not easy. If you do not attain the highest level it is because the energy was severed during issuing, making everything uncertain and obscure. This is certainly not the behavior of a spirited man.

Formerly Yang Pan-hou used this type of issuing on an opponent. He was able to make both of the opponent's feet leave the ground, and with one advance he could throw the opponent back about thirty six feet. Contemporaries considered this skill of Yang's to be the highest excellence. His father, Yang Lu-chan, on the contrary regarded it as incorrect. He reasoned that correct issuing energy must contain the characteristics of interrupting and frozen energies. The mind must be at peace and empty of offense. To issue you must be ingenious and utilize mind-intent.[3]

Beyond this there is still shaky springing energy. When yours and the opponent's energy no longer sticks together, then use the energy of the waist and legs to use shaky patting energy on him. Both of the opponent's feet will be raised off the ground and moved back. The response could also be that the hand strike (patting) will knock him directly to the ground like a bounced ball. Even more uncanny is that the initial pat repels him downward. Next, there is the issuing of long energy. After the opponent issues, you can then bounce him as though repelling him upwards. This is a very profound and abstruse energy.

Except for borrowing and drilling energy, all the other energies prior to issuing must have neutralize, entice and seize. When you have first obtained a good position you can only then speak of issuing. Otherwise it will be ineffective to just issue. This is the difficulty of having a beginner's coarse sensitivity. After thoroughly understanding one energy, you can completely comprehend all the other energies. If you don't possess the essence of any one energy, you will be unable to satisfactorily make use of any of the other energies.

The training of issuing energy is a prerequisite to your learning. You should first know the energy routes. Taking the body as a whole for example, where are the roots? Where are the branches? Where are the leaves? Where are the roots, branches and leaves in the upper portion of you body? Where are the roots, branches and leaves in the lower body? Now, in the body as a whole the root is in the feet, the trunk is the branches and the head, the leaves. In the upper body, the shoulders are the root, the elbows the branches and the hands, the leaves. In the lower body, the legs are the root, the knees the branches and the feet, the leaves. Therefore, in seizing or issuing to an opponent you must first subdue their root.[4] This is called, "to go up into the hall and enter the inner chamber." Correctly said: "to defeat an opponent, first break his root." When you fully comprehend the meaning of this, then and only then can you issue to an opponent. Otherwise you are, "climbing a tree to hunt for a fish" (a waste of time) and you will in the end acquire nothing.

When initiating issuing energy to an opponent there must be three essential points present: *opportunity, direction,* and *timing.*

"Opportunity" is putting yourself in a position where the opponent's back is turned and his center of balance is leaning to one side, thereby revealing his center point (*chiao tien*). In other words, when the opponent's center of balance is completely aslant, there is one place on his upper body where you can issue quite simply.[5] (This is the one place where they can be broken off from their root). Their ch'i will rise upwards simultaneously.

"Direction" refers to the tendency of the opponent's force, whether moving upwards or downwards, left or right, cardinal or diagonal. Whatever the direction you must follow and go towards their back when turning, and then issue.

"Timing" is that moment, just in the nick of time, when the opponent's old energy is exhausted and his new energy has not yet come out. You can then issue quite simply.

At the time of withdrawing you cannot go too soon or too late. If you withdraw too soon the opponent will not complete his movement which can easily lead to the defect of resistance. If you withdraw too late, it allows the opponent, having already revealed himself, to change his position.

Not one of these three can be deficient. Knowing

the *opportunity*, but not knowing the *direction*, will make it easy for the opponent get rid of all resistance when you attack, or that you mistakenly create the defect of resistance in yourself. Knowing the *opportunity*, but not knowing the *timing* will make it easy to resist your attack or have you make the mistake of insufficient issuing. All three of these must be intact if issuing to an opponent is to be done with ease. With the ease of a pill rolling off your hand, you will succeed in every endeavor. If your issuing power is fierce, yet you do not know how to employ it in accordance with the above three points, then it is just a lot of talk.

Besides these three points you must also pay attention to the distance between you and the opponent. If you keep too far away you cannot reach them and penetrate. If you are too close your energy becomes obstructed and weakened, and you will be incapable of issuing energy.

When issuing energy high or low, or upwards and downwards, there are also these relationships to be considered. If the opponent goes high, you must go high; if the opponent goes low, you must go low. If the opponent goes too low, you can then issue to their upper body; if the opponent goes too high, you can then issue to their middle or lower body. Additionally, you must pay close attention to whether the opponent's body is tall or short, big or small, light or heavy.

Generally, issue to the upper body of a short person, and issue to the middle or lower portion for tall people.

To the greatest extent possible issuing should be directed at the middle of the body whether they be tall, short, light or heavy. But if tall and light or short and heavy your issue should be directed at their lower body; if tall and heavy or small and light your issue should be directed at their upper body. To distinguish their lightness or heaviness during *t'ui shou*, use adhering and sticking energy, or enticing and neutralizing energy.

The exact place to issue is sometimes directed to their substantial part, and sometimes to their insubstantial part. This makes it impossible for them to make any changes to these parts. There are also times when the fingers entice out their force and then your palm issues. In summary, insubstantial to insubstantial; substantial to substantial. First, destroy and confuse the opponent's sense of bearing, entice their center point out and then issue. Follow the opponent's crouching down in order to take advantage of his bent position. So, if the opponent crouches, follow his crouching and then issue; if the opponent bends, follow the bending and then issue—always making use of their positioning and force by following.[6]

At the highest level of skill, your center point is very small and subtle, yet when issuing the opponent's center point is seen as very big [apparent]. As for which part of the opponent's upper body you should select, anywhere will be suitable for enticing out his center point for issuing to. Likewise, any one part of your body can equally initiate an issue to the opponent, yet this issuing must take place in the minutest fraction of time—entice and then issue. This will cause the opponent to be amply startled and out of position. At the time of issuing you must also seek to make the entire body move as one unit, and not be caught unawares when going out to issue.

Even if the opponent lacks energy I am still very perceptive of myself when issuing. When I am the subject of issuing I am still very perceptive and sink heavily. On the other hand, if the opponent's outgoing energy is quite fierce, you must be perceptive. For in being attacked, and to actually not receive it, is the real substance of the central theory. Within this theory there are certain particulars: there are those who perceive their energy, but their issue relies on being substantial. The energy will then by no means completely pass through and out. There are those who are perceptive, but lack the energy—being too passive the energy passes out and comes to an end. Therefore, issuing energy must be like shooting an arrow—*seeking the straight within the curved*—then the energy will come out completely. Do not cause it to stop short within the hands and arms, by extending them out too much when issuing.

When issuing you must adapt your body to performing the principles of keeping the *wei lu* centered and upright; retaining a light and sensitive energy on top of the head; hollowing the chest and raising the back; sinking the shoulders and suspending the elbows; seating the wrists and straightening the fingers; neither straighten nor bend the arms too much. (The internal energy completes a large spherical shape, just like *threading through nine crooks of a pearl*). Simultaneously, cause the backbone to slightly protrude and seat the waist and the entire perineum area. This is similar to the effects of a gun recoiling from a shot bullet. Only in, *seating the waist*, you must not consider this as moving to the rear, because in moving to the rear you will cause the energy to draw in or coil to the back and this will make it impossible to issue to the front.

Within issuing energy there are two applications for the internal circulation of the ch'i. One is by way of *the before going to the after*. There is a common saying, "from the *hsien t'ien* (before heaven) the *hou t'ien* (after heaven) is moved." This is the ch'i sinking into the tan t'ien. The ch'i is drawn out by way of the tan t'ien and passes through the four limbs. The other is *the after going to the before.* There is a common saying, "from the *hou t'ien* the *hsien t'ien* is moved." This is the ch'i adhering to the spine and arms. The ch'i is compelled out by way of the spine and arms and passes through the arms and legs.

The energy of issuing to an opponent is in one instance like throwing something. Wanting to throw something will result in throwing, but you cannot be divided about this. The slightest hesitancy in wanting to throw, will cause you not to throw. Because this will make you anxious, the mind-intent and ch'i are then easily severed. Once the mind-intent and ch'i are severed, how can you issue to an opponent? Therefore, when issuing to an opponent you must gather the ch'i and concentrate the spirit. The eyes should be fixed on the opponent, on no account gaze off somewhere else, otherwise in trying to protect yourself you may be knocked down. Gazing off somewhere else will also make the energy move downwards.

It is said in the *T'ai Chi Ch'uan Classic*, "Looking upwards, it seems to become higher and higher; looking downwards, it seems to become lower and lower." It is then said, "it is necessary to know the place of the spirit," as mind-intent and ch'i follow each other, even when energy is being issued. Mind-intent and ch'i cannot afford to be severed. This is called, "even if the energy is severed, the mind-intent is not severed." For if the mind-intent becomes severed so will the spirit.

The highly skilled are able to follow the neutralize and to follow the issue. They maintain small circles, the skill of which becomes ever deeper and ever smaller. They take half a circle to neutralize and use the other half to issue. Because of this, the style is not ordinarily seen. This is called, "advancing is withdrawing, and withdrawing is advancing; drawing in is letting go, and letting go is drawing in."

This story was previously handed down during the time of Yang Chien-hou. One day he was sitting inside his courtyard, inhaling the smoke from his tobacco pipe. Right before this a disciple had hastily requested further instruction. So Yang ordered the disciple to strike his stomach with his fist full force, and the disciple brought down his fist directly. Yang immediately let out a smile and then a loud *ha!* In one instant he made his stomach like a drum and the disciple immediately stumbled and fell into the outer courtyard. Yang resumed sitting, quietly inhaling the smoke as if nothing happened. His disciple afterwards was confused about what kind of energy it was that he was subjected to that could throw him so far away.

Yang Chien-hou's eldest son, Yang Shao-hou, when residing in Nanking, happen to meet up with a mad dog on the road one day. The dog attacked his legs,

but during the moments the dog was coming in, but
had not yet reached him, Yang used his knee, bending
it down just once. The dog was then turned and sent
out several tens of feet. This was definitely the highest
form and most profound use of issuing energy. This
also reveals the absolute ingenuity of his spirit.

Notes:

1. *Fa* is comprised of three radicals. The main radical, *po*, originally meant to turn your back on or not to follow. Hence, to disagree. The lower left radical, *kung*, represents a bow. The lower right radical, *shu*, an arrow. Therefore, the character *fa*, originally meant to shoot an arrow at an enemy, and has come to mean, "any expansion of a latent energy." From this comes the ideas of issuing, to send forth or to manifest.

2. *Red* in Chinese thought represents both good fortune and/or blood. So the verse here can really mean either, "when I strike with my hands, I will achieve a good result" or "...I will see my opponent's blood."

3. It is well-known that Yang Pan-hou, Yang Lu-chan's eldest son, had a very harsh temperament, and that his father had a very mild nature (as had Chien-hou, his second son). The obvious contrast here in deployment of issuing energy is yet another example of these differences in character. Yang Lu-chan's view does express a much higher understanding of issuing. Instead of expending the energy of throwing an opponent back thirty or more feet, Yang simply stopped the opponent dead in his tracks, interrupting and freezing his actions and intent. Furthermore, Lu-chan obviously understood the ingenuity of having no mind or intent of fighting, "at peace and empty of offense."

4. When thinking about defeating an opponent in t'ai chi ch'uan, the first object of attention is to destroy the opponent's root. Here is a description of how to locate that root. If the opponent's entire body is coming at you, then you must attack his substantial foot to destroy his root; if the

opponent attacks you by striking with his arm, you must go to his shoulder to destroy the root of his force; if the opponent attacks you by kicking, you must obstruct his opposite leg or seize his kicking leg to destroy the root.

Within t'ai chi ch'uan issuing methods, there are the principles of first seizing upper, middle and lower. In brief, *lower* means that your leg must attach itself to the opponent's leg to destroy his root, in one manner or another, as there are several; *middle* means that your issuing hand attaches to the back side of the opponent or in his mid body area, which then issues up and out to the opponent's body; *upper* means, that the other hand has seized the opponent's wrist, elbow or shoulder (depending on the circumstances and posture) to apply a forward and downward oblique pulling or enticing intent. When an opponent is subjected to all three simultaneously it proves rather difficult to remain standing.

5. This is a reference to what is normally called *lines of issuing*. "Lines" are in general, points and directions of issuing to an opponent, which takes the least amount of energy to fell an opponent. Lines are probably the least known of all t'ai chi ch'uan techniques and skills. This probably stems from the fact that unless a student has developed some skill with some of the basic energies, lines cannot be applied effectively anyway. The use of the line is the true meaning of the verse in the *T'ai Chi Ch'uan Classic*, "four ounces removing one thousand catties." It is the use of these lines which makes the push of a t'ai chi ch'uan master look so effortless, as though there was some magical or mystical energy at play. Indeed not, just good physics. There are according to Master Tung-tsai Liang, twenty-five lines which his teacher, Prof. Cheng Man-ch'ing claimed to know. However, Liang admits he only managed to learn ten

of these from his teacher.

6. This means, attach to the insubstantial aspects of the opponent's body with insubstantiality; attach to the substantial aspects of the opponent's body with substantiality. For instance, if the opponent's left side is empty, then just attach to it, but don't try to issue to it; the right side is full (resistant), then feint a push to get his breath up and extending him off his center. See note 4 of *Enticing Energy*.

7. The obstacles of the upper body and lower limbs are joints subject to seize and can be made immovable. See note 2 of *Seizing Energy*. Briefly, the middle body obstacles are referring to the idea that ch'i (breath) can be held in the chest, which causes you to lose your center and if struck in the chest while filled with air could cause a lung to collapse; the abdomen can also be caused to resist and attacked with damaging consequences; if the tan t'ien is not kept under control then your entire being can be disrupted and confused.

Borrowing Energy
Chieh Chin

借
劲

*I*n t'ai chi ch'uan borrowing[1] is a very profound and high form of issuing energy. Those who are not highly skilled cannot put it into proper use. Because in borrowing energy from an opponent's issue, there is no need for enticing and seizing, there is also little need for neutralizing energy, as these are all hard to control and go too far for borrowing.[2] Just be in accord with the activity and issuing, do not add to the anxiety. If the opponent's actions are hurried, then move fast like the wind or lightning. Take advantage of the opponent's force by borrowing his strength. If they come in high, move high; if they come in low, move low. Then it will not be necessary to focus on the view of going against his strength, and you will be able to use your opponent as he comes at you and catch him unawares.

This energy also has a rarer meaning: if an opponent comes in and then you move away, or if the opponent comes in and you then move towards him, their in-coming strength will be greatly increased, causing them to become the object of an attack with a very fierce energy.

The Song of Pushing Hands states, "to remove a thousand pounds with the momentum of four ounces." This is borrowing energy. The purpose of borrowing energy is for a smaller force to defeat a larger force. To yield means the counter-attack is then stronger. To be skillful at this method you must, in any event, be capable of changing, so that you can completely borrow from the opponent from any position and be able to issue to any part of their body. Yet when issuing to the opponent make sure the waist and legs act as one unit; sink the shoulders and suspend the elbows; hollow the chest and raise the back; keep the wei lu centered and upright; and use the mind-intent and ch'i when issuing.

You must also take into account the timing, as you cannot be either early or late. If you are early and the opponent's energy has not yet gone out, what then can you borrow? If you are late you will fall into a trap and be unable to act. The most opportune timings are when the opponent's energy is just about to come out, but is not completely out; or, when it is about to reach its end, but has not completely arrived. Then, within a split second, issue and you will have a good result. This is as if your opponent was about to put a foot inside the door of your house and you suddenly slam it shut on him. He would then have no way in which to get inside. Another reaction to this could be the door knocking him away and the opponent letting out a shout. Wait for him to open his mouth to shout and then seize him. When you seize his mouth by laying your hands on him you obstruct his ch'i and cut short his shout. From these examples you can know the training and practice of borrowing energy. These truly are not easy to do or to spontaneously put into practical use. In t'ai chi ch'uan this is called the highest vehicle.

The above transmission is a type of issuing energy. Within the Yang family the father and sons could bring forth this energy. This then is borrowing energy.

Notes:

1. The main radical of *chieh* is *jen*, meaning people, person
or persons. On the right side is *hsi*, which originally meant
dried meat, as the character depicts meat hanging in the
sun, and later developed into meaning "old days," probably from the idea of old dried meat. From the incorporation
of these two images, comes the meaning of "people of former days." In the present we avail ourselves of their wis-
dom, knowledge, experience and ancestry—hence to
"borrow."

   Borrowing energy is in theory very simple, in application very difficult, because it depends on how skilled you
may be with all the other energies. The clearest way of
explaining this would be through the analogy of supposing
a very large ball, suspended from a rope, were swung at
you from a distance. When the ball approaches your body,
you must first adhere your hand to the side of the ball, turn
your waist and step to the side simultaneously and then
push the ball off into the same direction it is going, giving it
even a greater force of momentum. If the ball were an
opponent and borrowing energy was applied to him, the
sensation would be that his very outgoing force increased
and so fell completely through and beyond his target.

   Another manner of looking at borrowing energy is to
suppose you are pushing an opponent and he resists
through being heavy to root into his feet. Feel immediately
for this resistance and just as immediately let go of it and
immediately again issue to him in either diagonal direction.
In this sense you are borrowing the reaction force of his
meeting with no resistance. As he attempts to regain his sta-
bility you simply issue to him. This is also an excellent test
of root. Many t'ai chiists have seen, heard or read of a t'ai
chi ch'uan master letting multiple persons push on them

simultaneously without their ability to push him over. This is genuine root if those pushing let go quickly and the person is still standing upright and centered. But it is not genuine root if they stumble forward or struggle to keep their balance, which means they were merely resisting you with their upper body to keep upright. Genuine root is in the waist, legs and feet, not the upper body.

In conclusion, to borrow means you must give back. Therefore, this energy should always be thought of in terms of receive and attack, withdraw and attack, as borrowing is within all of these providing that the opponent's strength or force is used against him.

2. Borrowing is much more refined in application than enticing, seizing and neutralizing. Therefore, in comparison, these energies are more difficult to apply in the context of returning energy to an opponent. This is not meant to take away any importance or need of enticing, seizing and neutralizing—borrowing is so distinct that there is no need of these other energies.

Opening Energy
K'ai Chin

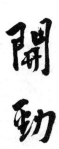

*T*he activity of opening[1] is in observing the entrances. Observe the moment of the opponent's in-coming energy to neutralize and open. There is opening energy and then the direction of that energy, along with the development of your mind-intent. Employ this energy to penetrate the opponent's inner entrances. If the opponent's strength is unusually resolute, this is the opportunity to use the body and stepping methods, as each of these are joined and related to each other. In trying to be distant from the opponent you will create the defect of maintaining a distance; which makes it impossible to employ the technique practically.

When opening you must make use of the energy of the waist and legs, in addition to mind-intent and ch'i. By no means use just the hands and arms. Even if there is sufficient force in the hands and arms to open, it would be foolish and dull-witted to attempt it. To achieve the appropriate standard for applying open to an opponent, the timing must be precise and the issue immediate. An error here causes your energy to become easily severed and all the positive results of the application will be lost. This deficiency will create the opposite result of the opponent being able to take advantage of the situation. In summary, if seeking to open the opponent's back so that you are presented with a good opportunity, make sure to stop at that point. Having obtained a superior position from opening, you can then directly affect the opponent's body and follow your own intentions.

Only the highly skilled can open these entrances often and naturally with just their mind-intent. Be cunning: as the opponent advances to enter, wait for him to enter deeply into your trap, then seize the opportunity to counter-attack. This is the method of "returning and giving."[2] Which is also in harmony with Lao Tzu's statements, *"in wanting to obtain something, you must first give,"* and; *"all thieves steal in the same manner."* But suppose the thieves have not yet entered your house, by what means can you catch them? Wait until they have entered, and when they are just about to steal your things, then capture them. How easy and fittingly just this is in the end!

Opening energy is contained within the framework[3] of *thirteen posture boxing*.[4] But its applications are numerous, including, *lifting hands, white crane spreading its wings, withdraw and push*, and many other. Even experienced students tend to think that these are just spontaneous workings.

Opening energy, even without interpreting or neutralizing, can still be issued to an opponent. This issuing, however, must contain the mind-intent of ward-off. Therefore, after opening, there must be an issue. If there is no issue, you will lose your opportunity.

Notes:

1. *K'ai* is formed by two radicals: the main radical is *men*, meaning a door, gate, an opening or entrance; the other is *ch'ien*, meaning to raise with both hands, level and even. The idea is then the image of opening a gate equally and evenly with both hands.

   Since the ideas of opening and closing are intrinsically tied together, further commentary on opening has been placed under *Closing Energy* (the following section).

2. Actually the idea is closer to "return what has been given," or, "give back what has been received." Usually this is referred to as "receive-attack" energy. When an opponent gives his energy to you (attacks you), then you give it back to him. This is much like pushing down on a metal spring, only to have it immediately spring back at you when your hand is taken away. So if an opponent pushes on you, then absorb about seventy percent of his force, directing it all into your rear foot and then issue it back to him. This method is even more effective if you initially apply receiving or borrowing energy, as these will make the issuing even stronger.

3. *Pan chia tzu* is a very broad term in definition, but "framework" will do for the most part. However, this term is meant to express not only the roundness of the posturing, but the individual gestures within the postures themselves, along with all the pertinent principles to be applied.

4. "Thirteen posture boxing" (*shih san shih ch'uan*) is an earlier and alternate name for t'ai chi ch'uan.

Closing Energy
Ho Chin

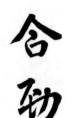

The opposite of opening is closing.[1] A common verse says, *"one yin and one yang."* With every opening there is yang; with every closing there is yin. If there is an opening, there must be a closing. Hence, these two words, opening and closing, share a very close relationship to one another. Therefore, departing brings about closing. So if an opponent tries to get away, take advantage of this and perform close.

Closing is a circular energy, and also has the mind-intent of being near and joining together with the opponent. During the time of closing use the energy of the waist and legs; sink the shoulders and suspend the elbows; hollow the chest and raise the back; and, adhere the ch'i to the back of the spine. In the postures of *thirteen posture boxing*, this energy is seen in *lifting hands, playing the guitar, withdraw and push* and *conclu-*

sion of t'ai chi, which all have the mind-intent of closing energy.

In t'ai chi ch'uan closing energy is very, very
important. The closing energy intention is strongly
present when issuing energy. It is able to bring forth
the body's whole ch'i. The focus of closing and issuing
is to completely defeat the opponent. This is the reason it says in *The Mental Elucidation of the Thirteen
Kinetic Postures,* "Direct the ch'i, as if threading the
nine crooks of a pearl, penetrating between every
minute crevice." This means, at the time of issuing
energy that all the closing ch'i should go out like the
striking of a drum, just like closing the *nine crooks of a
pearl* in one action. Without this issuing energy, the ch'i
cannot congeal. If it cannot congeal it will disperse and
the issuing will have no good result.

Notes:

1. The character for *ho* means harmony, to join, to agree and to close or shut. The main radical here is *k'ou*, which simply means the mouth or talking. The image above this is *chi*, which consists of three lines, forming a union of three people (or many). Hence, the idea of a group in agreement or a harmonious closing of a discussion.

The ideas of closing are expressed in the classics in various manners, such as: In the *Song of the Thirteen Postures*, it says, "Whether bending or stretching, opening or closing, listen and let them take their natural course." Bending means to draw in, like a bow ready to release an arrow; stretching means to issue, to shoot the arrow.

Here are some of the dialectics for the terms of opening and closing:

Opening	Closing
Adhere	Issue
Inhalation	Exhalation
Adhering the ch'i to the spine	Issuing the ch'i from the spine
Raising an opponent's ch'i	Issuing to the opponent's ch'i
Making the opponent defective	Seizing the opportunity
Rising	Sinking
Adhering	Sticking
Receiving	Borrowing
Raise the back	Hollow the chest
Receive	Attack

In *The Mental Elucidation of the Thirteen Postures* it says, "First seek to be open and expansive; after seek to be close and compact."

In the *T'ai Chi Ch'uan Treatise* the defects of opening and closing are expressed as, "Avoid deficiency and excess; avoid projections and hollows; avoid severance and splice." The defects associated with opening are: *deficiency, projections* and *severance. Excess, hollows* and *splice* are the defects of closing.

The most difficult concept to initially understand is the example given in *The Mental Elucidation of the Thirteen Kinetic Postures*, "Direct the ch'i, as if threading the nine crooks of a pearl, penetrating between every minute crevice." The imagery of *nine crooks of a pearl* has various meanings. First of all, *threading* is opening and *penetrating* is closing; the *pearl* is your body. Externally these nine crooks refer to nine joints on the body in which the ch'i and energy must pass through in order to issue: the ankle joint, the knee joint, the hip joint, sacrum area, scapula areas, shoulder joint, elbows joint, wrist joint and finger joint (knuckles). If any of these joints or areas are defective, there is then an obstruction, and neither the ch'i nor energy can move freely through them. This would be similar to the thread breaking. From the feet to the fingertips, all must be relaxed for energy to be released and opened in order to direct the ch'i.

Internally the *nine crooks* refer to two *Tao yin* exercises. 1) The ch'i is visualized and directed through nine cavities in order to complete either the Small Heavenly Circuit or Larger Heavenly Circuit. (See Chapter Four, *Cultivating the Ch'i, Volume One*.) 2) The ch'i is directed to each of the nine apertures, using the techniques of sealing (*closing*) and releasing (*opening*). The nine apertures are: the two eyes, the two ears, the two nostrils, the mouth, front yin opening (urinary tract) and rear yin opening (anus).

Rising Energy
T'i Chin

提
勁

Rising[1] is referred to as, rising to draw up. In t'ai chi ch'uan this energy has one purpose, to adhere. You use your energy to draw up an opponent in order to uproot him, which causes him to lean off his center of balance. He stumbles over and his posture is destroyed. This is certainly easier if I originally make myself heavy and then rise up and become light. It will be quite difficult on the other hand if I am incapable of applying this skillful method. This skillful method is to take advantage of an opponent during the time he is unawares. Move forward with advance step and using the energy of the waist and legs, rise upwards and adhere. This will cause the opponent to be caught unawares, to be defective, and to lean off his center of balance.

To achieve rising rely entirely on the waist and

legs. Do not use the hands for rising. To use the hands for rising makes you heavy and clumsy. It is quite easy for an opponent to perceive your issuing. Therefore, when rising the feet must be firmly rooted; relax the ch'i into the tan-t'ien; retain a light and sensitive energy on top of the head; adhere the ch'i to the spine; keep the *wei lu* centered and upright; gather the ch'i and concentrate the spirit. Focus the gaze firmly on the opponent. There must be a great resolve in order to root up a mountain or to rise to its peak.

Beyond this you need to take into account an opponent's direction, distance, and use the body and stepping methods. This is particularly true when you respond to an opponent's convergence. You may still be connected to him, but you will achieve no gain from it. In practical application you follow to seize your opportunity and respond by adapting to the changes.

When you obtain a good position from rising, you must then also entice. It will not matter which energy is used, as all of them are capable of issuing an attack. There is then no opponent which can not be sent away. This energy's intention is explained in the *Song of Pushing Hands*, "Entice the opponent to advance, then let him fall on emptiness, adhere and then issue." Students who are not highly skilled in rising energy, cannot be accomplished. Instead of taking advantage of the opponent's emptiness and then entering, they try to be clever and so completely fail. Students must pay heed to this.

Notes:

1. *T'i* derives its meaning from *shih* (on the right side), what is controlled by the sun's light, and by *shou* the main radical, which means, the hand or to support. Thus, the idea of "supporting that which is controlled by the sun's light," which is growth. So by extension the idea of growth developed into rising, as all life does.

Rising energy is intrinsically bound with the energy of sinking. The classics refer to them in a dualistic manner, just as with opening and closing, but not always in terms of rising and sinking. For example, in the *T'ai Chi Ch'uan Treatise*, it says, "... upwards and downwards ... are to be directed by the mind-intent, and not to be expressed externally." It also says, "If the initial intent is upwards, you must first have a downward intent. If you want to lift something upwards, you must first have the intent of pushing downwards." Upwards and downwards are aspects of rise and sink. Therefore, "rise and sink are to be directed by the mind-intent" and "If the initial intent is to rise, you must first have a sinking intent. If you want to raise something, you must first have the intent of sinking." There can be no rising without the intent of sinking, and no sinking without the intent of rising.

A minor defect of rising is to bend forward; of sinking is to lean back. The *T'ai Chi Ch'uan Classic* states, "Do not incline and do not lean." However, the major defect of rising is double-floating and of sinking, double-weighting. This classic also says, "Sinking the weight to one side results in adapting to circumstances. Double-weightedness results in being impeded." By extension here it could also be said, "Not sinking the weight to one side results in not being able to adapt to circumstances. Double-floating results in being impeded." Therefore, excessive rising leads to double floating, and excessive sinking leads to double-weighting. Which is why there can be no rising without the intent of sinking, and vice versa. For further discussion on double weighting and floating, see text of *Sinking Energy* and note 5 of *Receiving Energy*.

Rising is *yang* and sinking is *yin*; rising is inhaling and adhering the ch'i to the spine, and sinking is exhaling and sinking the ch'i into the tan t'ien; rising is bringing the opponent's ch'i and root upwards, sinking is to keep your ch'i and root downwards; rising is coming up off the rear leg to issue, and sinking is draw in the *wei lu* to keep centered and upright; rising is advancing, and sinking is withdrawing; rising is expanding, and sinking contracting; rising is to draw up, and sinking is leading down, and so on.

So in the *Song of Pushing Hands*, as quoted in this section, "Entice the opponent to advance, then let him fall on nothing, adhere and then issue," which precisely refers to the idea of enticing an opponent upwards or forwards (advance or rise). Entice him to rise and then immediately sink so that he has nothing to hold onto, then adhere (stay lightly attached with his falling off) and issue when he begins losing his center of balance.

Sinking Energy 沉
Chen Chin 勁

Opponents regard sinking[1] and heaviness as one in the same. They really are not! Heaviness is visible and sinking is invisible. Heaviness is a non sensory and obstructive force. Sinking energy is lively and appears relaxed, but is not so relaxed; appears tense, but is not so tense.[2] Sinking is assuredly not the same as heaviness.

When a student is doing *t'ui shou*, they will for the most part be unable to distinguish clearly the differences in an opponent's sinking and heaviness; or their lightness and floating. With each of these it is easy to unwittingly get side tracked. The original authors (the Yang family) scrutinized these, purposefully revealing the proper meaning of these four words.[3] The full details are given here so that those who practice may have a short cut in which to follow in their footsteps and understand the true path.

Partially light and partially heavy is not a defect; being completely light or heavy is a defect. "Partially" means there is defined positioning; being "complete", there is no defined position. If you are complete, without a defined position, you lose the square within the circle.[4] If you are partial, with a defined position, you do not lose the square within the circle.

Partially sinking and partially floating is a defect, because it is inadequate and insufficient; completely floating or sinking is a defect, because these are excessive and deficient.

Being partially or completely heavy is a defect because you are impeded and cannot advance. Being partially or completely light is a defect because you are nimble, but have no circularity. To partially or completely sink is a defect because there is insubstantiality, with no offsetting substantiality. To partially or completely float is a defect because they are without spirit and not circular.

What do you suppose could come after these? In comparing the actions of floating and double-lightness, neither can advance—from these come lightness and nimbleness. In comparing the actions of heaviness and double-sinking, neither can advance—from these come distancing and insubstantiality. These two are the very best.

In summary, internally you must be light, nimble and not confused; externally the ch'i is clear, bright and capable of being sent throughout the body and limbs. This is the beginning of the correct method.

The ability to sink and issue this energy, will cause an opponent to be sent flying. This is because the ch'i goes out from the tan t'ien through the spine, arms and hands, and then penetrates into the opponent's body. This causes him to soar as if jumping back. This is like striking a ball extremely hard, so that it bounces up very high. This energy is very fierce and within the issuing energies is one of the most important.

It is said in the *T'ai Chi Ch'uan Treatise*, "If the initial intent is upwards, you must first have a downward intent. If you want to lift something upwards, you must first have the intent of pushing downwards. Then the root will be severed; it will be immediately and certainly toppled." This quotation is the gist of this whole energy. Students must pay heed to this.

Notes:

1. *Chen* carries the meaning of perishing, of heaviness and something sinking into the water. The main radical is *shui* (on the left) and means water. On the right side is *yin*, which originally meant to go away or withdraw. Hence, *chen* came to mean something withdrawing into the water, sinking. See section and notes on *Rising Energy*.

2. These statements are derived from the *Song of Pushing Hands* and *The Mental Elucidation of the Thirteen Kinetic Postures*, where they state, "Appearing relaxed, but not relaxed." They also derive from the *T'ai Chi Ch'uan Classic*, "To suddenly disappear and suddenly appear." These verses are easily misinterpreted by t'ai chi*ists*. What appears to make the body look relaxed is *sung*; what makes it not so relaxed is energy. What *suddenly disappears* is *sung*; what *suddenly appears* is energy. *Appearing relaxed* is external, and *not so relaxed* is internal; *suddenly disappearing* is external, and to *suddenly appear* is internal. The *T'ai Chi Ch'uan Classic* also says, "Yin is not separate from yang; yang is not separate from yin." Again, like rising and sinking, energy cannot be separated from issuing; withdrawing cannot be separated from advance, and so on. Likewise, if there is to be *sung*, you must first have the intent of issuing energy. Meaning, if there is to be *sung*, there must first be the intent of "non-*sung*;" if there is to be suddenly disappearing, there must be the initial intent of suddenly appearing, and vice versa. By analogy, the cat watching the rat may look relaxed externally, but is very active and alert internally. Also, only ten percent of your t'ai chi ch'uan movement is actually seen externally, as ninety percent of the movement takes place internally. See note 3 of *Listening Energy*.

3. These four words are: sinking (*chen*), heaviness (*chung*), lightness (*ching*) and floating (*fou*).

4. The square in the circle is a very broad concept of t'ai chi ch'uan principle and theory. Here it is referring to the principle of movement. In t'ai chi ch'uan there are postures and within the postures there are individual gestures. Each of these gestures are the defined movements of the waist and legs, which get you from point A to point B. In performing a posture you have a beginning stance and an ending stance—all the movements to connect those are gestures. These gestures follow the eight directions, four cardinal and four diagonal. These are the *square(s) within the circle*, which then also apply to all posturing, whether solo or two-person.

Ward-Off Energy
Peng Chin

棚
勁

*I*n *t'ui shou* ward-off[1] energy is extremely important. If you were without ward-off energy when engaged in *t'ui shou* you will need to practice non-resistance to overcome the opponent. Do not use the hands and arms in applying ward-off, you must use the waist and legs, in addition to mind-intent and ch'i. This will make it very difficult for the opponent to both enter and attack. This is the method of protecting.

In seeking to issue to an opponent, before ward-off there must be an initial action towards the back and down. Use enticing energy to induce him, cause his energy to come out and to seemingly provide a focal point for him. Make use of his energy and ward-off. Then you can be victorious. If not, you must empty the opponent's strength and make him insubstantial. Otherwise there will be no way in which to borrow and you will be unable to use ward-off.

It is best to position yourself, in ward-off, where you place your opponent's joints in a position where you can break them.[2] Because, in doing this, the opponent finds it quite difficult to escape.

In seizing the opportunity when the conditions for ward-off come about, you must quickly issue an attack. If not, all your efforts of going "to and fro" will be in vain. Then what meaning is there?

When there is ward-off and issue you must gather the ch'i and concentrate the spirit; focus the gaze firmly on the opponent. If you are doing ward-off to the east, yet gazing off to the west, there can then be no good result.

Notes:

1. *P'eng* is a specialized character, not found in the Chinese dictionaries. *P'eng* was originally pronounced as *feng* and represented the tail feathers of the mythical bird, the phoenix. By the inclusion of *shou*, the hand, the meaning of grasping a bird's tail came about. Indicative to Yang style only, the postures of *grasping the bird's tail*, left and right styles, have presently come to embody the postures of ward-off (*peng*), roll-back (*lu*), press (*chi*) and push (*an*), which all have the appearance of different forms of "grasping a bird's tail." But for sake of clarity, originally in the Yang style *p'eng* represented only ward-off, and *lang ch'ueh wei*, a more literal manner of saying "grasping a bird's tail" were in fact two totally distinct postures (left and right styles).

The original order of performing the Yang style postures was: 1) *Beginning posture of t'ai chi ch'uan* 2) *Grasping the bird's tail, right* 3) *Grasping the bird's tail, left* 4) *Ward-off* 5) *Roll-back* 6) *Press* 7) *Push*, and so on. This posture order must have been changed I suspect with Prof. Cheng Man-ch'ing's arrangement of his short form. In his form, the number of total postures are abbreviated by counting *ward-off, roll-back, press* and *push* as one posture, calling it "grasping the bird's tail" (or in his view, "grasp the sparrow's tail") and through eliminating the right style of the two styles of "grasping the bird's tail," he had redesigned the opening order and number of postures. In Chen style t'ai chi ch'uan however, the style Yang Lu-chan had learned previous to inventing his own family style, there is no reference to any posture called "grasping the bird's tail;" but in the Wu style, created by Yang family disciple Wu Chien-chuan, "grasping the bird's tail" does appear.

With ward-off the explanations of all eight postures

begin. They are: *ward-off, roll-back, press, push, pull, split, elbow-stroke* and *shoulder-stroke*. With the inclusion of (the five activities) *advance-step, withdraw-step, look-left, gaze-right* and *central equilibrium*, the thirteen postures are formed. The "five activities" are not, however, in any sense postures, but rather *posturings* which are contained within each of the eight postures and are thus not associated with energy.

In the treatise *Secrets of the Eight Postures* it says,

"What is the meaning of ward-off energy? It is like a boat floating on the water. Sink the ch'i into the tan t'ien, then suspend your head from above. The entire body acts like spring-like energy, instantly opening and closing. Even if confronting one thousand catties, you can uproot and cause the opponent to float without any difficulty."

2. This means to initially bring the opponent's arm in close to your body, so that the back of his elbow is attached to your body and his wrist is seized by your hand. This will obstruct and make his shoulder, elbow and wrist immovable. It also appears like someone holding a large bird in their arms.

Roll-Back Energy

Lu Chin

掤
劲

In roll-back[1] one hand is placed near and adheres to the opponent's wrist; your other hand and forearm sticks along the opponent's arm; and when your body reaches the rear, you roll-back. In this way you assist the opponent's insufficient issuing energy. When issuing energy, many opponents will fall off as they move towards the back of you. It's as if you already knew the opponent's weak point. His center of balance will be brought leaning to the front, making it impossible to move back and look up. The right opportunity to employ roll-back is to take advantage of his forward leaning, then entice and do roll-back. Make use of his forward leaning and falling off when your body is moved to the rear. Most certainly this skill would be shallow and useless without adhering and sticking energy. For it is easier to be the object of an opponent, so as to take advantage of his faults and directly enter.

There are those who possess adhering and sticking energy, but they may not necessarily have accomplished this method of roll-back. Likewise there are many who cannot subdue nor control an opponent. There are two reasons for this. *One* is the inability to entice an opponent previous to roll-back. You must first have the intention of ward-off energy, as ward-off will initially cause the opponent to resist. Only when there is this resistance, can you roll-back. *Two* is the lack of understanding about the proper direction of roll-back. Many beginning students will just use straight lines when trying to apply roll-back. The highly skilled, having both the body and stepping methods, certainly have the capacity for this energy. But if expert skill is not refined, then you can do no better than apply diagonal lines of thirty degrees to either the left or right, which is the best. With the energy of the former it is easy to be the object of slipping off. The latter is similar to borrowing the energy of the opponent. Performing roll-back to an opponent is similar to moving the catch of a lock. It is entirely in the waist and legs, mind-intent and ch'i, and not in the hands and arms.

As you begin your roll-back, your waist and legs should rise up slightly until the ward-off reaches the front of the chest, and when the time is right with the opponent's back to you, then seat the waist and relax the coccyx, turn the waist, roll-back and issue to him. If you are too excessive with any of these techniques you will be unable to issue and to knock him over. Excessiveness will only exhaust your strength. Your issuing will then also lack ability, and your lack of a good position will compound the problem.

When you roll-back and issue, integrate your spirit and vitality; focus your gaze firmly on the opponent. Then the opponent will fall, but you must maintain your gaze without any faltering. This is what is meant in the *Mental Elucidation of the Thirteen Kinetic Postures*, "The energy may be severed, but the mind-intent is not severed."

In *t'ui shou* roll-back energy is extremely important. If you cannot roll-back, you cannot make your opponent bend over to the front. Still less, you'll be unable to move and shift his center of balance. It will be difficult indeed to be victorious.

Notes:

1. *Lu* is another specialized character invented by the Yang family, which translates as "roll-back." This character is formed through the combination of three ideograms. *Shih*, pertaining to positions of the body; *fu*, to return; and, *shou*, the hand. Hence, the idea of returning the hand. In the past many translated this as *pull-back*, which hardly bears any resemblance to the actual posture instructions given within the explanations of the solo form.

The idea of roll-back, in one instance, comes from turning the palm upwards and over the hand of the opponent, a rolling over and back gesture. But this must be done with lightness, not with force. Force will just create the opportunity for the opponent to continue the direction of force and come around to strike you. The best position is to adhere lightly to his wrist area, with your thumb attached to the back of his little finger. Then there is nothing to counter against. On the other side your elbow must stick to the opponent's elbow, which allows you to not only deflect his whole energy, but also to set up a lock on his elbow joint for a possible break.

The above allows you to readily either seize, receive, borrow, entice or issue, and will greatly improve your ability to adhere and stick, listen and interpret. Afterwards, the internal functions of roll-back will be seen in rising, sinking, opening and closing.

This particular posture and concept was, without doubt, one of Yang Lu-chan's greatest additions to t'ai chi ch'uan, and there are many others as well. The roll-back posture is also only found in the Yang style of t'ai chi ch'uan, it does not appear in Chen style or Wu style. However, this particular posture is so extensive and highly refined in the Yang style system that mastery of it will literally mean that fifty percent of your t'ai chi ch'uan development is mastered. Roll-back is a neutralization and so plays an intrinsic part in every application. In the solo form postures, all the gestures within a posture, except one (issuing), are for the most part designed to neutralize and lead the opponent off his center, which are the functions of roll-back. Those who practice *san shou* and *ta lu* will readily understand the importance of roll-back in every posture. Whether you are the object of any of the other seven postures, it takes roll-back, in one form or another, to neutralize it.

In the treatise *Secret of the Eight Postures* it says,

"What is the meaning of roll-back energy? Entice the opponent to advance forward, follow his incoming energy, do not discard it nor resist it. When his strength is completely exhausted, he will naturally be empty. At this point you can let go or counter him. Maintain your own center and no one can take advantage of you."

For further discussion on neutralize and roll-back see note 3 of *Neutralizing Energy*.

Press Energy
Chi Chin

Press[1] entails using your lower forearm to press and strike the opponent's body. In *t'ui shou* this movement is one of the most important. But you cannot go too high or too low. Press happens after your roll-back. Therefore, the conditions must be satisfactory when considering press. First fully complete your intended roll-back, then change and press your opponent.

Press can also be used after an opponent's shoulder-stroke. Only this press does not use hand or arm strength, rather the energy of the waist and legs is used, appropriate with the ch'i and mind-intent. The manner in which to respond to his shoulder-stroke is by completely rounding out and not moving into a slanting position. Suspend the head and keep the body upright; sink the shoulders; hollow the chest; draw in the *wei lu*. Do not bend the upper body forward, to avoid falling off your center of balance.

If you use strength to press, it will only serve to make it easier for the opponent to counter to your forearm and borrow your energy. The highly skilled are able to press effectively by uniting it with the ch'i, causing the opponent to turn his back [a defective posture] and thus restricting his whole body.

When issuing this energy you can make use of long, sinking and intercepting energies. Beginning students of *t'ui shou* consider that it is to a greater extent defective to press with just one hand within the *four hands*[2] exercises. Therefore, their circling in *t'ui shou* is not very rounded. It is the rare student who pays full attention to this.

Notes:

1. *Chi* means to crowd, to squeeze or to push against. A common phrase in Chinese describing someone in dire straits is *chi shou*, to press the hands together. This character is built upon these two radicals, *ch'i*, to be even and level and *shou*, the hands. Hence, the idea of pressing the hands together.

Press is performed differently within the styles of t'ai chi ch'uan. Even in Yang style there are two main variations. In one the left hand palm is attached to the inner forearm, with the left and right elbows positioned like ward-off posture. In the second variation the left hand fingers are placed onto the right wrist, with the left elbow hanging down and the right elbow and arm positioned at about a thirty degree slant. Each of these are correct, it is only a matter of discretion and application as to which one is used. The first one, which is the traditional Yang style manner of performing press, is used to press the opponent's body, making use of long and sinking energies. The second one, seen in other forms of t'ai chi ch'uan, but popularized by Prof. Cheng Man-ch'ing, is used to press the opponent's cavities. It is a very quick and sharp type of press and makes use of intercepting energy.

In the treatise *Secrets of the Eight Postures* it says,

"What is the meaning of press energy? It functions in two ways. 1) The simplest is the direct method. Go to meet [receive] the opponent and then adhere and close in one action. 2) To apply reaction force is the indirect method. This is like a ball bouncing off a wall or a coin tossed onto a drumhead, rebounding off with a ringing sound."

2. These are the applications of *ward-off, roll-back, press* and *push* performed as a repetitive exercise, both on a horizontal

level plane and vertical circular manner, as well as in a
fixed step and active step manner.

Push Energy
An Chin

按
劲

*I*n push[1] an opponent can be pushed with either one hand or both.[2] In order to push you must go with the stepping to obtain a good position. Otherwise, it will not be easy to do. In push there is the mind-intent of opening and closing.[3] Maintain a perpendicular circle when moving forwards or backwards. If the push is hard and straight, its function is already lost. Then the situation will be reversed and you will fall victim to your opponent.

When you open and close in push, your hands and feet must correlate whether advancing or withdrawing, whether raising or falling. Stepping and rising are insubstantial; a falling step is substantial. The insubstantial creates the conditions for entice; the substantial creates the conditions for issuing. To do push you must use the energy of the waist and legs, along with appropriate ch'i and mind-intent. Focus your gaze firmly; retain a light and sensitive energy on top of the head.

You cannot move away too quickly, as being too quick will to the contrary make it easier for the opponent to borrow your energy. If the opponent is able to take advantage of your waist and legs when you extend forward, your arms will collapse and crumple when pushing out. The opponent will certainly be aware of your difficulty and be able to restrain you.

When pushing it is necessary to suspend the head to keep the body upright; sink the shoulders and suspend the elbows; hollow the chest and raise the back; seat the waist and relax the coccyx; draw in the *wei lu*; do not bend the upper body forward, as this will cause your center of balance to come forward, which makes it much easier to be rolled-back and out. Make sure you pay attention to this.

When pushing an opponent, the highly skilled regard true energy for the most part as something which occurs before you issue. You must put yourself in a good position, with the opponent's back exposed, automatically causing them to either bend, look up, jump up or stumble back.

Within the issuing energy of push there are also the

divisions of long, intercepting and sinking energies. Additionally, you must understand the practical application, adapt to circumstances and then act.

Notes:

1. *An* means to place the hands on, to press down (as in massage) and to restrain something from moving. It is formed by the two radicals of an, to be peaceful, quiet, natural and without effort; and shou, the hand. We have the image of hands that are at ease, or of doing something with the hands effortlessly. The idea of push, as defined in English, is really not expressed here in the Chinese. But then rightly it should not be expressed, for the idea of pushing something embodies the idea of force and an is an issuing energy, which is an expression of effortlessness of the hands, and push is actually issued by the waist and legs, not the hands. The *T'ai Chi Ch'uan Treatise* says, "The energy is rooted in the feet, issued through the legs, directed by the waist, and appears in the hands and fingers." This clearly shows that the hands are only the expression of a push, appearing like a push, which really came from the foot. It is from this appearance that the translation of an into push came about, simply because it looks like the hands are pushing.

In the treatise *Secrets of the Eight Postures* it says,

"What is the meaning of push energy? When mobilizing this energy it is like flowing water. The substantial is concealed within the insubstantial. The force of a torrent is difficult to oppose. Reaching a high place, it swells and fills the entire space; coming into a low place it descends into it. There are troughs and crests within waves; there is no opening into which they cannot enter."

2. This is called, "yin-yang pushing." If you are faced with an opponent who has no *ch'uan* skills, he can be pushed with both hands because he knows nothing of neutralizing nor of substantial and insubstantial interplay. In other words, he is all clumsy or brute force. However, if you are

confronted with someone who does have *ch'uan* skills, then you must push with one hand only, so not to be trapped by meeting with no resistance. One hand could be used to entice the opponent while the other hand actually pushes; or, one hand pushes while the other waits in reserve in case the other hand is neutralized, then that hand can be used for push.

3. See sections on *Opening Energy* and *Closing Energy*.

Pull Energy
Ts'ai Chin

ull[1] is the grasping of the hand, wrist or elbow of an opponent and then by moving down to sink and pull. The function of this is very similar to roll-back.

Right at the time when you are just about to make the opponent come forward and off his center of balance, you then take advantage of this opportunity and make him fall forwards. But this kind of pull is without the use of the hands. Pulling with the hands only makes the outcome less beneficial. You must use the energy of the waist and legs, with appropriate ch'i and mind-intent.

Pull implies attaining a good position by confusing your opponent, and making him dizzy. His whole body and heels must be raised when pulling. When both heels are raised, you can then issue to him. But in pulling an opponent, do not attempt to pull both sides. Only one side must be pulled, because then you can make the opponent's center of balance lean in one direction. If not, then you will become the object of the opponent's borrowing energy and stable center of balance.

Now, in pulling an opponent you cannot pull too lightly, as lightness makes it easier for borrowing to be done to you. There would then be no reason to pull, as it is already being done to you. So when pulling, you must pull sufficiently. This yields a comparatively greater result.

When pulling your entire body must be centered and upright; sink the waist and seat the legs; hollow the chest and raise the back; sink the shoulders and suspend the elbows; sink the ch'i into the tan-t'ien; and, the focus is directed downwards.

In the *T'ai Chi Ch'uan Classic* it says, "Looking upwards, it seems to become higher and higher; looking downwards, it seems to become deeper and deeper." Within *thirteen posture boxing*, the posture of *needle at the sea bottom*, is the method and application for pull. *Needle at the sea bottom* is followed and connected to *fan penetrates the back*, which is then followed by the intention of issue.

Notes:

1. *Ts'ai* means to pluck, gather, choose and within t'ai chi
ch'uan terminology, to pull. The character *ts'ai* is built on
three ideograms. The first is *shou*, meaning the hand; second, *mu* for wood or a plant; the third is *chao*, which means
to grasp. Hence, picking flowers or plants with the hand,
pulling.

    In t'ai chi ch'uan texts, pull is usually discussed right
along with push. For example, in the *T'ai Chi Ch'uan Treatise*
it says, "If you want to pull something upwards, you must
first have the intent of pushing downwards." In the *Mental
Elucidation of the Thirteen Postures* it also says, "When you
push and pull, withdraw and attack, your ch'i adheres to
the back of your body and is gathered into the spine."
Pulling is an uprooting technique, just as push is. In both
cases, they are considered successful when the two feet are
caused to leave the ground, obviously in different manners.
In pull the opponent falls forward and down obliquely; in
push the opponent falls straight back and upwards. Pull
destroys the root of the opponent by bringing him *deeper
and deeper*; push destroys the root by bringing him *higher
and higher*. In regards to applying the technique of affecting
lower, middle and upper, pull affects the upper body of the
opponent by pulling his upper torso diagonally downwards; push (the middle) issues to the opponent's torso.
From these examples it is easy to see the importance of
pull.

    In performing pull, there are four main principles
which must be adhered to: 1) Attach your pulling hand
unto the opponent's wrist only after having enticed him
downwards with sink. 2) Once the opponent follows your
sinking, attach your hand to his wrist in the same way that
a baby grabs at your finger, firm and yet without the tens-

ing of the muscles. 3) After sinking into your front leg and you are attached to the opponent's wrist, turn diagonally away and down in a whipping like action, which will cause both of his feet to rise and his body to topple forward and down. 4) Immediately withdraw into your rear leg and let go of the opponent as soon as he begins falling forward, or help him along further by pushing on his back with your opposite hand. So, when pulling, shift into your front leg; when being pulled sink into your rear leg. For another example of how pull works with t'ai chi ch'uan kicks, see Chapter Six, section four, *Ts'ai Tui Method*, in *Cultivating the Ch'i, Volume One, Chen Kung Series*, by Stuart Alve Olson. Dragon Door Publications, 1993. Also, see note 5 of *Issuing Energy*.

In the treatise *Secrets of the Eight Postures* it says,

"*What is the meaning of pull energy? It is like weighting a steelyard beam. No matter how substantial or insubstantial the force is, the heaviness and lightness of it can be clearly distinguished. To push or pull requires but four ounces, yet a thousand pounds can be balanced by it. In asking what is the principle of this, the answer lies in the function of the lever.*"

Split Energy
Lieh Chin

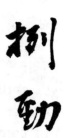

Split[1] energy is not used very much in t'ai chi ch'uan. Those who know of it are very few. It is not as familiar as the energies of ward-off, roll-back, press, push, pull and shoulder-stroke. You should become experienced with this energy, as it is truly very important. Students should be aware of this energy. For instance, when you have placed your opponent in a defective position and he is bending forward or leaning back, be in accord with his turning out. You must then turn and use this energy. His energy will then be unable to react.

The energy of split is used after roll-back or pull. To apply split, one hand pushes on the opponent's arm; use the back of the other hand by turning it over and leading the opponent into split. This will cause the opponent to look upwards, bend forwards, and then fall down.

If an opponent uses *parting wild horse's mane* on you and you end by looking up with your back exposed, then you can use split by turning and being in accord with his position, causing him to look up and lean back. As the highly skilled would put it, "In what manner is it absorbed? In what manner is it returned?" When the opponent tries to make me lean back and stumble, I then take this leaning and stumbling and return it to him.

Split is divided into the methods of *horizontal-split* and *pull-split*.[2] But each must make use of the energy of the waist and legs, and not the hands. Also, when using this you must pay attention to the distance between you and the opponent. You cannot be too far apart, as being too far apart will not give you a good result. So, you should properly use the body method and stepping methods to properly converge with your opponent—then you can achieve a good result.

Beyond this you still need to always guard your interior entrances.[3] Otherwise in trying to be clever you will completely fail. Certainly, the opponent, will then take advantage of the opening and enter.

Notes:

1. *Lieh* is another specialized character invented for the posture of split. The character shows a hand (*shou*) holding a sword (*Tao*) which is cutting (*tai*), Hence, the idea of splitting.

Splitting makes a great deal of use of the legs, in either causing the opponent to fall over the leg placed behind his front rooted leg or in sweeping away the foot while performing split to the upper body, a scissors like action. So the idea of split has a great deal to do with "cutting away" at the opponent's root.

In the treatise *Secret of the Eight Postures* it says,

"What is the meaning of split energy? Like a spinning disc, if something is cast onto it, it will be immediately thrown out more than ten feet. Have you not seen a whirlpool? The rolling torrent and spiraling currents; if leaves should fall in they are quickly dragged down it and disappear."

2. *Horizontal-split* is used in the *san shou* and *ta lu* sets, where the back of the forearm comes across the upper body of the opponent, the opposite hand seizes the opponent's elbow and the front leg steps behind the opponent's front leg. Then using the waist and legs, turn slightly to cause the opponent to fall back and down. Another example of horizontal-split is to seize and issue to the wrist and elbow, making them immovable, after roll-back. *Pull-split* can be seen in the execution of *needle at sea bottom* (pull) moving into *fan penetrates the back* (split). But the main uses of pull-split lie in the applications *diagonal flying* and *playing the guitar*.

3. "Interior entrances" (*nei men*) are the mental functions—your mind-intent, ch'i and spirit—which can be confused,

distracted, angered or made fearful. Guarding these interior entrances is a matter of sinking the ch'i into the tan t'ien, focusing the gaze and concentrating the spirit.

Elbow-Stroke Energy
Chou Chin

肘
勁

*E*lbow-Stroke:[1] When an opponent strikes with his hand (the fingers, palm, fist or wrist included) your reaction should be to keep it away from your body. But trying to keep it away can actually make it easier to clash with the hand even before it fully arrives. This is the defect of your energy being already severed. Trying to be too near also can impede your maneuvering, and you will be unable to issue. When you use your hands to prevent this defect of being either too separated or too close, you are unable to achieve a superior position. Then only elbow-stroke can help you.

There are two things to consider when applying elbow-stroke: The hands are less effective than the elbows for attaining a good position to issue. The elbows are more brutal than the hands, because you can strike directly into the pit of the stomach, a most aggressive move.

When issuing unite the knees, using the energy of the waist and legs, along with appropriate ch'i and mind-intent. Your whole body must be upright and straight; retain a light and sensitive energy on top of the head; hollow the chest and raise the back; sink the shoulders and suspend the elbows; draw in the *wei lu;* focus your gaze firmly on the opponent.

These are also the essential conditions within *ta lu.* Elbow-stroke is found in roll-back when you bring your elbow around and strike your opponent. In *t'ui shou,* elbow-stroke is found when separating to open the opponent's hands. One hand grasps the opponent's hand, the other arm employs elbow-stroke to his mid-chest region.

This energy is very fierce. If you attempt to use it, without acquiring the correct method, your opponent may well borrow on you. Therefore, when using this energy pay special attention.

Notes:

1. *Chou* does not translate purely as elbow-stroke, in fact stroke is not even implied by the character, but as the entirety of the forearm, from the elbow down to the wrist. *Ju*, the main radical, means the fleshly areas above the wrist (the forearm to the elbow); *ts'un*, means inch and comes from the primitive meaning of a dot, which represented the place on the wrist where the pulse was felt, which is about one inch from the hand. To translate this as elbow-stroke is very much an implied meaning, based on the function of the posture rather than the ideogram itself.

In the Yang style solo form of t'ai chi ch'uan you will not find a posture named elbow-stroke, as it is contained within the posture of *chop with fist*, and there are several variations of elbow-stroke within these. The general idea is that "elbow-stroke" and "chop with fist" are applied with the intent of "folding up" energy. This type of energy comes from the ideas expressed in the story of how Chang San-feng invented t'ai chi ch'uan while watching a magpie attacking a snake. In brief, when the bird struck at the snake's head, the tail whipped up to strike the bird; if the bird attacked the tail, the head darted up to counter the bird; if the bird attacked the middle of the snake's body, both the tail and head came up to attack. In human beings this translated into, if an opponent grasps your fingers, the wrist attacks; grasping the wrist, the elbow strikes; if seizing the elbow, the shoulder strikes; if the shoulder is seized, the head attacks. Further, if the right side is attack, the left side counters it, and vice versa; if the upper is attacked, the lower part strikes, and vice versa; if the middle is attacked, both arms of the upper body attack (i.e., *push* and *strike with both fists*).

In the treatise *Secrets of the Eight Postures* it says,

"What is the meaning of elbow-stroke energy? The function is in the Five Activities. The yin and yang are distinguished according to upper and lower. The substantial and insubstantial are to be clearly discriminated. If its motion is connected and unbroken, nothing can oppose its strength. The chopping of the fist is extremely fierce. After one has thoroughly understood the six energies,* the functional use is unlimited."

*The six energies are adhere, stick, neutralize, seize, entice and issue.

Shoulder–Stroke Energy
K'ao Chin

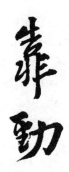

S houlder-stroke[1] entails bringing the shoulder to shoulder-stroke the mid-chest area of the opponent. This posture is also like elbow-stroke, and is very severe. It is used when your body is at a distance from the opponent and you are positioning to get near him. When you are the object of closing and you are unable to issue energy, use the assistance of elbow-stroke.

During shoulder-stroke keep your whole body centered and upright; unite the hips and shoulders. But you cannot bring the tip of the shoulder to collide hard with the opponent's body. When you and the opponent come together you must simultaneously touch his skin slightly, use your energy of the waist and legs, with appropriate ch'i and mind-intent, and shoulder-stroke him.

Whether high or low, follow to seize the opportunity and then act. The correct placement and stepping is to make sure you pay close attention to the steps and enter by going to the inside of his trouser leg, creating a T-shape. If not, then you will be unable to obtain a good position.

The applications for shoulder-stroke in *ta lu* are very numerous. Therefore, students find this very easy and clear. Yet, when performing shoulder-stroke you must retain a light and sensitive energy on top of the head; hollow the chest and raise the back; keep the *wei lu* centered and upright; focus the gaze firmly on the opponent. Then the opponent will simply be knocked over.

Beyond this, you must be able to protect your face when shoulder-stroking in case the hands or arm when shoulder-stroking are flung up. For once there is a quick separation, it will be easy for the opponent to strike your face or even break your arm. Therefore, in doing shoulder-stroke one hand must be ready to protect, the other arm bends and adjusts to do shoulder-stroke.

Guard against the unexpected, because shoulder-stroke may cause the body to lean somewhat, which will quite handily assist your opponent's attacking force. The shoulder's energy, is much greater than the hand or elbow's.

Notes:

1. *K'ao* means to lean against, and that is as close as the term gets to the idea of shoulder-stroke. The character originally meant to rebuke the wrong doings of another, but why the meaning changed is unknown.

Like elbow-stroke, you will not find a posture in the Yang style solo form called "shoulder-stroke," both these names are reserved for the *ta lu* and *san shou* exercises. The shoulder-stroke posture is however a transitional gesture from *lifting hands* into *white crane spreading wings*. Again, we don't see the actual posture name of shoulder-stroke appear in the Yang style until Prof. Cheng's introduction of his short form. In the Wu style of t'ai chi ch'uan we do not see any references to a shoulder-stroke posture. The founder of Wu style, Wu Chien-chuan, was a student of the Yang family. Chen style, the style Yang Lu-chan learned before inventing his own family style, does however have three elbow-stroke type postures within the *pao tui* (cannon fist) set, and one shoulder-stroke posture, *bend back to shoulder-stroke*.

In the treatise *Secret of the Eight Postures* it says,

"What is the meaning of shoulder-stroke energy? The method is divided into the shoulder and back techniques. In diagonal flying posture the shoulder is used, but within shoulder-stroke there is some use of the back. Once you have the opportunity and positioning, the technique is like the pounding of a pestle.
Pay attention to your center of balance. If you lose it, the technique will be in vain."

Long Energy
Ch'ang Chin

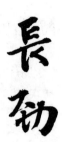

This energy[1] is both soft, gradual,[2] and very elongated. In application any and every part of the opponent's body will do: the hands, arms, elbows, shoulders, waist, thighs, knees, legs and feet.

Having enticed and neutralized the opponent during *t'ui shou*, gradually bring your energy to extend out and issue to any of the above focal points on the opponent's body. But suppose that after neutralizing, the opponent still manages to reach you and you are unable to repeat another neutralize. Your positioning must then be turned out, as if to meet and obstruct your opponent's energy. Your energy must then yield and bend in advancing to the front. Follow his posturing, without discarding and without resistance, advancing when there is an opening. In these situations, it is like as *threading through nine crooks of a pearl.*

Yet if the energy applied is too great the thread will break and you'll be unable to advance. If the energy is too little, you will have trouble converging and you will be unable to advance. Without following the gestures of bending and curving, it will be impossible to thread through with any skillful energy.

It is said within *The Mental Elucidation of the Thirteen Kinetic Postures*, "Direct the ch'i, as if threading the nine crooks of a pearl, penetrating between every minute crevice." This is one way of explaining it.

When issuing you must sink the shoulders and suspend the elbows; keep the *wei lu* centered and upright; use the energy of the waist and legs, with appropriate ch'i and mind-intent.

When using long energy, or perhaps initially using intercepting energy the highly skilled will blend in long energy. If you initially use long energy and the opponent is about to come out with an attack, yet does not really come out, you can then catch him with intercepting energy. First intercept, then use long energy. This will cause the opponent to first shrink back. When the opponent withdraws and the long energy is completed, you then turn out. First long, then intercept, makes the opponent initially turn and then shrink back, allowing the energy to be issued. So before entering or afterwards when going away from the opponent's body, always gather up and unite your energy. First enter, then leave. For example, springs extend out to become very long; but if the coil still has some slack, it can become even longer. It can extend out very quickly and it can also recoil very quickly. But even without this slack, it is not completely exhausted even at its end. This long energy is a wonderful mystery of t'ai chi ch'uan. Those who practice t'ai chi ch'uan should never be caught unawares by long energy.

Notes:

1. *Ch'ang* has various meanings like long in duration, to increase, to excel and old. The character is its own radical and in the primitive meant a piece of hair so long that it needed to be tied to a brooch. From this came the idea of becoming a man (older).

   In the *T'ai Chi Ch'uan Treatise* it says, "With every movement string all the parts together, keeping the body light and nimble." *Stringing all the parts together* is sometimes presented in the analogy of a long string of pearls strung together, so that when one pearl is moved, they all move according to the initial motion. Long energy must be continuous and connected, as it is a soft and gradual energy. This same classic also says, *"Ch'ang ch'uan is just like a long river or great ocean rolling on without interruption."* Long boxing is another, older name for t'ai chi ch'uan. It was called *ch'ang ch'uan* because its movements were soft, gradual and long, like a river's current flowing on ceaselessly. In *The Mental Elucidation of the Thirteen Postures* it says, "move like a river current ... mobilize the energy just like reeling silk." When reeling long pieces of silk from a cocoon it must be done gradually and softly, otherwise it will break and be of no use. These verses from the classic were chosen here to not only demonstrate how intrinsically important and fundamental long energy is to t'ai chi ch'uan, but to clearly point out that this energy is the norm for t'ai chi ch'uan. This is stated because when you truly have *sung*, anxiety and hurried reactions are left far behind. Because of this, when sparring or being attacked, the movements of the opponent do not seem as fast or quick as they would if you were full of anxiety and tension. This is just like when we were small children, summer vacation, even a normal day would seem to last forever, because we had no real anxiety and tension. It isn't until we get older that life becomes rushed, shortened and full of anxiety. So long energy is like a very playful and gradual manner of turning, yielding, bending and so on, until the entrance or crevice is found in the opponent's defenses. This is also why long energy is equated with "threading nine crooks of a pearl," which must be done softly, gently, slowly and gradually.

2. *Jou* means equally to be soft, pliable and gentle; *man* means equally to move gradually, continuously and slowly.

Intercepting Energy
Chieh Chin

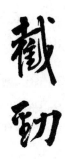

nother name for intercepting energy[1] is hard energy.[2] In application any and every part of the opponent's body will do: the hands, arms, elbows, shoulders, waist, thighs, knees, legs and feet. The practical function of this energy rests entirely on enticing the opponent to meet with no resistance. Just at the moment he is becoming aware of this and unable to change or neutralize, follow this with issuing to his center. His posturing then will become hurried and over-anxious, and the force of the attack and the falling back he is subjected to will be very fierce.

When this energy is issued you must suspend the head with a light and sensitive energy; hollow the chest and raise the back; sink the shoulders and suspend the elbows; keep the *wei lu* centered and upright; gather the ch'i and concentrate the spirit; use the energy of the waist and legs, with the appropriate ch'i and mind-intent; keep the gaze focused firmly on the opponent. Then the opponent will most certainly be knocked down.

When issuing this energy, there are two types, an arc line and a straight line,[3] followed by the application of the posture used. Beginning students when acquiring this method and wanting to put it into use, will assuredly find it to be no easy matter.

Notes:

1. *Chieh* means to cut into two, to obstruct, to cut off and intercept. The character shows a bird (*chui*) being completely and equally (*shih*) cut in two by a lance (*ko*). Hence, the idea of intercepting or cutting off an opponent's energy. However, do not confuse this intercept with that of the posture, *step forward, deflect downward, intercept and punch*, as that intercept (*lan*) has a closer meaning to parry than does *chieh*. These are not the same.

This type of energy, in function, causes the opponent through enticing to react prematurely to an anticipated issue, at which point the intercepting resembles an opponent being thrust back as though lanced by a spear. No sooner than the opponent is searching to regain his center of balance he is met immediately with intercept. The opponent can be met with using either the torque-like (arc) or straight line applications from any of the postures.

2. *Kang* means, hard, unyielding, vigorous and diamond-like. It is called "hard energy" because the opponent feels as though he ran smack into a brick wall and as a result is repelled back, stunned and confused.

Drilling Energy
Tsuan Chin

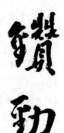

rilling[1] is an entering energy, employing the use of either the fingers or fist. It is used when first coming into contact with an opponent's skin. Then as if drilling into wood, enter with a circular torque-like action. This energy is very resolute and the strike can cause serious injury to the opponent's internal regions.

When you apply this energy hollow the chest and raise the back; sink the shoulders and suspend the elbows; retain a light and sensitive energy on top of the head; and, sink the ch'i into the tan-t'ien. Entirely apply your mind-intent and all your ch'i when issuing this energy. This energy can also completely destroy an opponent's *nei kung* (internal skill), just like the type of ch'i kung called, *pi k'ou kung* (closing the cavities skill).

In t'ai chi ch'uan this energy is really a specialized form of long energy, only the focal point and function are not the same. With this energy it is easy to injure an opponent. Beginning students should not necessarily attempt a thorough examination of this, so they may avoid seriously injuring others accidentally. Hence, the original text conformed to just a few words of explanation.

What is the training method for this energy and in what situation should this be issued to an opponent? Without an experienced and reputable teacher to orally give you the mind-transmission, you cannot know.

Notes:

1. *Tsuan* means, to bore into, to penetrate, to pierce and to drill. The ideogram is made up of *chin*, metal or gold; *tsan* which means to pay a visit or enter the home of another. Hence, along with the image of metal, *tsuan* came to mean, to drill or bore into.

This energy is very dangerous. But unless the attacker knows the exact location of the seven fatal cavities on the human body and likewise knew the training methods of *pi k'ou kung*, there is not even a slim chance that it could be employed. The danger here is that beginning students, who have not received the transmission of this energy, will proceed with things like iron palm training and so damage the sinews, compromising their chances of acquiring this energy, which is far superior and more refined than the external training of iron palm. Besides, as the text warns beginning students, there is much to be learned about t'ai chi ch'uan other than just learning how to hurt others with drilling energy.

Lofty Towering Energy
Ling Kung Chin

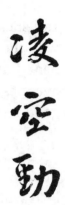

*L*ofty towering[1] energy is very different from the ordinary and even the mysterious. It actually approaches the mystical. You won't believe it unless you see it with your own eyes. Truly it is one of a kind. In function it is no more than a very superior spiritual energy.

The highly skilled, when issuing this energy, barely need to let out a *ha!* [2] sound from the mouth to remove the two feet of opponent off the ground and to repel him back. The goal of this issue is, to send out a spiritual energy which creates a power of attraction[3] that nothing can oppose.

Certainly, in order to issue this energy to an opponent you must first have an understanding of adhering and sticking and the other energies. Then afterwards, with the sensation of just one *ha!*, can repel your opponent. But without understanding the other various energies, trying to issue this energy will not have a good result.

Students seeking this energy, which is very mysterious and unfathomable, should not do so too intensely. It will certainly not suffice to just roam about looking for it.

Formerly this energy was transmitted by Yang Chien-hou's eldest son, Shao-hou. Through this power of attraction he was able to be about a foot away from a burning candle, and with one hand cutting across in front of the burning flame, extinguish it. This is of course just one method of lofty towering energy. Presently though, the transmission record of this kung fu has been lost.

Notes:

1. *Ling* means, to aspire, to rise, be pure and to be lofty. The ideogram is based on the two radicals of *ping*, which means the rays of light that rise up and appear through the crystallization of water when freezing and *ling*, which means a tumulus. Hence, many mounds or hillocks of crystallized light. *Kung* previously meant a cavern or cavity, but presently means emptiness, void or hollow. *Kung* is made up of two radicals *hsueh*, to bore into or cavern; *kung*, to labor.

2. See Chapter Three, *Internal Breathing Methods for Mobilizing the Ch'i,* Heng and Ha section, *Cultivating the Ch'i, Volume One, Chen Kung Series.* Compiled and translated by Stuart Alve Olson. Dragon Door, 1993.

3. *Hsi yin* literally means, to induce an inhalation. Thus, the idea of "the power of attraction." Here the meaning is expanded into a spiritual-mental power which cannot be resisted.

Afterword

*T*he above are the principle energies of t'ai chi ch'uan. Some of which are: sticking, receiving, enticing, neutralizing, seizing and issuing. But apart from these, there are still the energies of dispersing, twisting, breaking, grasping, inch, separating, playful shaky, folding up, along with wiping, peeling, deceptive, and approaching. The classifications are numerous, yet none of them are indispensable.

In summation: First, practice to develop your kung fu, by training to be compact, doing so until you obtain the knack of being compact. Then, going further, research the dimensions of the least proportions. From the foot to the inch; still further, from the inch to the tenth of an inch; still further, the tenth of an inch to the ten-thousandth part. Finally apprehend the minute fraction. You are then able to interpret, neutralize, seize and issue from any of the postures or gestures within t'ai chi ch'uan; or from any one of the styles of the *san shou* methods; or even from any acquired movements from the shaolin boxing school.

Each of these can be interpolated as is necessary. However, you must clearly distinguish the external gates from the internal gates, which have three stages of upper, middle and lower. Seize the good opportunities and obtain a good position. Follow the mind-intent and join the function. But it is not necessary to embrace just one style or method.

Those students who seek to acquire each energy, must thoroughly investigate to the very bottom of these matters, until all are completely understood. But even so, without receiving an oral mind transmission from someone highly skilled or from a reputable teacher, you cannot fully accomplish this end, as the original text barely explained the essential points.

An Explanation of Restraining, Seizing, Grasping and Closing

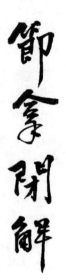

*T*he most profound mysteries of t'ai chi ch'uan are hardly found within the framework of the postures, *t'ui shou*, *ta lu*, *san shou*, saber, sword or even staff. In every energy there is an aspect of adhere and stick, neutralize and issue, nothing too much more can actually be said. But in former times there were these four types of kung fu: restraining, seizing, grasping and closing. Because the original principles of these were so very abstruse, it proved difficult for teachers to both transmit and train students. Consequently, up to the present day, the transmission is gradually being lost, as there is an unwillingness by teachers to part with it. The original text was not inclined towards detail and strategy, but contains some additional explanation. So, in general, it is necessary that every student is at least made knowledgeable of these.

Restraining means to restrain the blood vessels; *seizing* means to seize the meridians; *grasping* means to grasp the sinews, and; *closing* means to close the cavities.

If the *blood vessels* are restrained, the blood will not circulate or flow; if the *meridians* are seized, it will be difficult for the ch'i to move; if the *sinews* are grasped, the body will be without a commander or troops; if the *cavities* are closed, the vital principle will be no more.

If the blood does not circulate or flow, it is as if half dead; *if the ch'i does not move*, the body will look as ridiculous as a wooden chicken; *if the body is without commander or troops*, the strength is severed and dies; *if the vital principle is no more*, it will be difficult to stay alive.

When you have achieved this kung fu from the correct practice of *t'ui shou*, and your hands are able to sense the foot, inch, tenth of an inch and ten-thousandth of an inch, you will be able to measure an opponent. When you are able to measure an opponent you can restrain blood vessels, seize meridians, grasp sinews and close cavities.

Restraining does not necessarily require measuring, as it can also be acquired through push; *seizing* does not necessarily require measuring, as it can also be acquired through rubbing; *grasping* does not necessarily require measuring, as it can also be acquired through sensing; *closing* however cannot be acquired without measuring. Without measuring you will be unable to locate the cavities, as this type of kung fu requires the foot to shrink until it becomes an inch; the tenth of an inch to shrink until it becomes a ten-thousandth of an inch, and so on.

The human body has one-hundred and eight cavities. Seventy-two of them are not fatal and thirty-six can be fatal. Yet, there are seven of these cavities which can be instantly cut-off from ch'i, causing death. When these seven cavities are *closed*, it is as though the skin is set on fire. It is like entering a dream and receiving an awful fright. It can cause the bones to break and sinews to be torn away, or cause a violent and sudden death.

Now, in the event you come to understand the heart of this matter, it would be as if suddenly waking up and perceiving true nature. Because *closing* means to understand what is true, to know what is manifested, and to know what is the function of the spirit.

Afterwards you will be capable of entering the apertures, as if shooting an arrow. If you can understand that to be centered means not just adjusting the inclination of one side or correcting your angle, but rather in gathering the ch'i and concentrating the spirit, then everything will hit the mark! This is for the most part the conditions for closing cavities. Without a reputable teacher, you will be unable to receive a transmission of these four types of kung fu—*restraining, seizing, grasping* and *closing.*

The early masters were unwilling to propagate false teachings and did not trust just anyone. They were apprehensive about transmitting their kung fu skills to others without good reason.

Closing verse of the T'ai Chi Ch'uan Classic, attributed to the Immortal Wang Tsung-yueh.

The Principles and Essential Roots of T'ai Chi Ch'uan

1) *Retain a light and sensitive energy on top of the head.*

2) *Concentrate the line of vision.*

3) *Hollow the chest and raise the back.*

4) *Sink the shoulders and suspend the elbows.*

5) *Seat the wrists and straighten the fingers.*

6) *The entire body must be centered and upright.*

7) *Draw in the wei lu (tail bone).*

8) *Relax the waist and the entire perineum area.*

9) *The knees appear relaxed, but not so relaxed.*

10) *The soles of the feet must adhere to the ground.*

11) *Clearly distinguish the insubstantial and substantial.*

12) *The upper and lower parts must follow each other;
the entire body must act as one unit (once you move,
everything moves; once you are still, everything is still).*

13) *Unite the internal and external; the breathing must be
natural (inhale to inhale; exhale to exhale).*

14) *Use the mind-intent, do not use external muscular force.*

15) *The ch'i should circulate throughout the entire body;
dividing the activity into upper and lower (adhering it
to the back of the spine; sinking it into the tan t'ien).*

16) *The mind-intent and ch'i must be joined together.*

17) *All the postures and movements must be in agreement
with one another, do not separate or expose your back,
with the entire body comfortable and open.*

18) *All the postures must be uniform (neither too hurried
nor too slow); continuous and unbroken (externally the
postures are like this, and the internal energy and mind-
intent are also like this).*

19) *The manner of the movements must be without excess
and insufficiency; always seek to be centered and
upright.*

20) *Retain the functional use, but do not expose it.*

21) *Within movement seek tranquillity (a tranquil mind is without thought and without anxiety); within tranquillity seek movement (mobilize the internal ch'i).*

22) *Lightness begets nimbleness; nimbleness begets movement; movement begets change.*

Suggested Reading

T'ai Chi Ch'uan: For Health and Self-Defense - Philosophy and Practice
by Master T.T. Liang. Vintage Press, 1977.

Fundamentals of T'ai Chi Ch'uan
by Wen-Shan Huang. South Sky Book Co., 1973.

The Tao of Tai-Chi Chuan: Way to Rejuvenation
by Jou, Tsung Hwa. Charles E. Tuttle, Co., 1981

T'ai Chi Ch'uan and Meditation
by Da Liu. Schocken Books, 1986

Cheng Tzu's Thirteen Treatises on T'ai Chi Ch'uan
by Cheng Man Ch'ing. Translated by Benjamin Pang Jeng Lo and Martin Inn.
North Atlantic Books, 1985.

T'ai-Chi: The "Supreme Ultimate" Exercise for Health, Sport and Self-Defense
by Cheng Man-ch'ing and Robert W. Smith. Charles E. Tuttle, Co., 1967

T'ai-chi Touchstones: Yang Family Secret Transmissions
Compiled and Translated by Douglas Wile. Sweet Ch'i Press, 1983.

Tai Chi Ch'uan: The Technique of Power
by Tem Horwitz and Susan Kimmelman with H.H.
Lui.
Chicago Review Press, 1976.

Practical Use of Tai Chi Chuan (Its Applications and Variations)
by Yeung (Yang) Sau Chung. Tai Chi Co., 1976.

Lee's Modified Tai Chi for Health
by Lee Ying-arng. Unicorn Press, 1958.

Yang Style Taijiquan
Editor: Yu Shenquan. Hai Feng Publishing Co., 1988.

Wu Style Taijiquan
by Wang Peisheng and Zeng Weiqi. Hai Feng
Publishing Co., 1983.

Chen Style Taijiquan
Compiled by Zhaohua Publishing House. Hai Feng
Publishing Co., 1984.

Cultivating the Ch'i: Secrets of Energy and Vitality
Chen Kung Series - Volume One
Compiled and Translated by Stuart Alve Olson.
Dragon Door, 1993.

Imagination Becomes Reality: The Teachings of Master T.T. Liang
Compiled by Stuart Alve Olson. Dragon Door, 1992.

About the Author

S tuart Alve Olson began learning the Chinese language during his residency at the City of Ten-Thousand Buddhas in Ukiah, CA (1979-1980). In 1982 he was invited to permanently live in Master T.T. Liang's home in St. Cloud, Minnesota (the only student ever granted this honor). Staying with Master Liang for five years, Stuart studied both T'ai Chi Ch'uan and Chinese language under his tutelage. Since that time he has traveled extensively throughout the United States with Master Liang assisting him in teaching T'ai Chi Ch'uan. Stuart has also taught in Canada and Indonesia, and has traveled throughout Asia. He now lives in St. Paul, Minnesota where he teaches T'ai Chi Ch'uan, Taoist yoga and meditation at the Institute of Internal Arts, a non-profit organization he founded in 1992, and translates T'ai Chi books for Dragon Door Publications. He may be contacted through the Institute of Internal Arts, 253 East Fourth Street, Third Floor, St. Paul, MN 55101-1632.

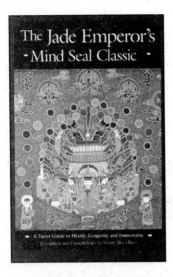

The Jade Emperor's Mind Seal Classic

A Taoist Guide to Health,
Longevity and Immortality

Translated by Stuart Alve Olson,
$10.95, paper, 128 pages,
15 illustrations
ISBN 0-938045-10-5

The Taoists believe that there is no reason for a person to ever suffer physical illness. Death itself, whether from old age or sickness, is an unnecessary occurrence. Illness and death occur as a result of the dissipation of the Three Treasures - ching, ch'i and shen - our reproductive, life-sustaining and spiritual energies. The secret science of restoring, gathering and transforming these primal energies creates an elixir which will confer health, longevity and immorality.

The Jade Emperor's Mind Seal Classic, presented here in the first English translation is a primer on how to achieve these benefits. A supreme distillation of Taoist thought, the text works as the catalyst for a deep transformation of the being.

Stuart Olson, Taoist practitioner and long-time protege of Taoist and T'ai Chi Ch'uan master, T.T. Liang, provides a lucid translation of, and an insightful commentary on this key text. With its wealth of practical information the commentary will further reward the reader with deeper insight into other great Taoist works, such as the *Secret of the Golden Flower* and *Taoist Yoga: Alchemy and Immortality*.

Olson supplements this classic with a further translation of a rare treatise on *The Three Treasures of Immortality* taken from the Dragon Door sect of Taoism. A collection of aphorisms and quotes from various Taoist scriptures and masters, *The Three Treasures of Immortality*, sheds further light on the processes that will lead you to enhanced heath and longevity, if not enlightenment and immortality.

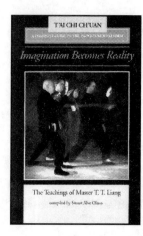

Imagination
Becomes Reality
The Teachings of
Master T.T. Liang

Compiled by Staurt Alve Olson,
$21.95, paper, 292 pages,
7"x11", 600 illustrations
ISBN 0-938045-09-1

T.T. Liang is one of the most revered living masters of T'ai Chi Ch'uan.
Now in his nineties, he has taught T'ai Chi for over fifty years. As a
senior student to Cheng Man-ch'ing and as author of the best-selling *T'ai
Chi Ch'uan for Health and Self-Defense* he helped introduce T'ai Chi to
America.

This book presents the very heart of Liang's teachings, including his own
version of the Yang style 150 posture solo form. Taken from T.T.'s own
notes, this is the most comprehensive description of the form ever presented. Rare interviews and articles by T. T. Liang explore the basic principles and meaning of this increasingly popular martial art.

The remarkable photography both captures the full power, grace and
subtlety of T'ai Chi while providing a detailed count by count presentation of each posture.

"Master T.T. Liang is a Chinese martial arts treasure in Western society.
He was a true pioneer in the development of T'ai Chi Ch'uan in the
United States of America."
    Dr. Yang Jwing-ming, author of Yang Style T'ai Chi Ch'uan

"This profound yet practical book...has much to offer practitioners of T'ai
Chi and those intrigued by the concept of heightened awareness."
    Australian Bookseller and Publisher

Cultivating the Ch'i
Chen Kung Series,
Volume One

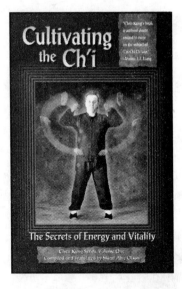

Translated by Stuart Alve Olson
$12.95, soft cover, 164 pages,
5-1/2" X 8-1/2,
101 illustrations,
ISBN 0-938045-11-3

Your foundation for health and
self-defense, this is the first English translation of a work considered by the Chinese to be the Bible of T'ai Chi Ch'uan.

Taken from the training notes of T'ai Chi's most famous family,
the Yangs, the book gives you detailed advice on breathing techniques, energy generation, meditation, ch'i-kung and much more.

You will appreciate the insightful commentary by Stuart Olson,
based on his own extensive experience as a T'ai Chi instructor.

"Chen Kung's book is without question second to none on the
subject of T'ai Chi Ch'uan."
          — Master T.T. Liang

"If you are interested in physical immortality, practice yoga, meditate or would like to explore a very ancient, revered and effective
way of maintaining physical vitality and youthfulness, you can
learn a lot from this book that you would simply never find else-
where."
          — New Age Retailer

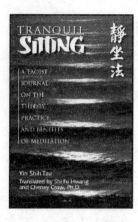

Tranquil Sitting
A Taoist Journal on the Theory, Practice, and Benefits of Meditation

Yin Shih Tzu
Translated by Shi Fu Hwang
and Cheney Crow, Ph.D.
8.5"x5.5", $9.50, soft cover, 128 pages
ISBN 0-938045-12-1

A modern Taoist Master's inspirational testament and practical guide to the healing power and spiritual benefits of meditation.

"Master Yin Shih Tzu's book so enthralled me that I read it in a single sitting. His training in classical Chinese medicine and as a professor of physiology enable him to express both his own experiences and his guide to cultivating a practice of these methods in a language easily comprehensible to the modern reader. His book is a wonderful contribution to our understanding of the nature of Taoist/Buddhist yoga, meditation, and inner science."
  Glenn H. Mullin, author of *Selected Works of the Dalai Lama* and *Death and Dying*

"The reader can really better understand the mental and physical phenomena encountered when progressing through meditation. If anyone ever wondered what changes may occur during intense study of mediation, this book helps to provide answers."
  Master Jou, Tsung Hwa, author of *The Tao of Tai Chi Chuan* and *The Tao of Meditation*

"This wonderful work has been very influential in my own practice and I was elated to find that Shi Fu Hwang and Cheney Crow had completed such a clear translation. *Tranquil Sitting* provides inspiration for all those who want to practice meditation, but may feel that their life contradicts or obstructs that practice. Yin Shih Tzu is deservedly considered one of China's most celebrated meditation practitioners."
  Stuart Alve Olson, author of *Cultivating the Ch'i*

Order Form

Name _____ Phone _____

Address _____

City _____ State _____ ZIP _____

Country _____

Title	Price	Quantity	Total Price
Cultivating the Ch'i	$12.95	_____	_____
Imagination Becomes Reality	$21.95	_____	_____
Intrinsic Energies	$12.95	_____	_____
Jade Emperor	$10.95	_____	_____
Tranquil Sitting	$9.50	_____	_____

Subtotal

MN Residents add
6.5% Sales Tax   _____

Shipping &
Handing ($3.00 for
first book, $1.00 for
each additional book.
Double S&H for
non-U.S. orders.)   _____

Totals   _____

❑ Check/Money Order Enclosed
❑ VISA   ❑ Mastercard
❑ Amex   ❑ Discover   Expires_____

Card #_____
Signature _____

Credit Card orders only: 1-800-247-6553
Dragon Door Publications
P.O. Box 4381, St. Paul, MN 55104 • ph. (612)645-0517

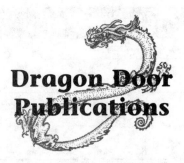

Dragon Door Publications

Dragon Door Publications also publishes a line of videos, audio tapes, and special reports and has a mail order catalog devoted to items on martial arts, meditation and Eastern philosophy. You may be especially interested in our three volume companion video to the book *Imagination Becomes Reality*.

Write, call or use our order form to receive a one year free subscription to our catalog.

Dragon Door Publications
P.O. Box 4381
St. Paul, MN 55104
(612) 645-0517
Fax (612) 644-5676